HOW TO LIVE A HEALTHY LIFE

D1339946

With best
wishes.

Books available from the same author:

By Appointment Only series

Arthritis, Rheumatism and Psoriasis
Asthma and Bronchitis
Cancer and Leukaemia
Heart and Blood Circulatory Problems
Migraine and Epilepsy
The Miracle of Life
Multiple Sclerosis
Neck and Back Problems
Realistic Weight Control
Skin Diseases
Stomach and Bowel Disorders
Stress and Nervous Disorders
Traditional Home and Herbal Remedies
Viruses, Allergies and the Immune System

Nature's Gift series

Air – The Breath of Life
Body Energy
Food
Water – Healer or Poison?

Well Woman series

Menopause
Menstrual and Pre-Menstrual Tension
Pregnancy and Childbirth

The Jan de Vries Healthcare series

Questions and Answers on Family Health

Also available from the same author

Life Without Arthritis – The Maori Way
Who's Next?

How to Live a Healthy Life

A Handbook to Better Health

Jan de Vries

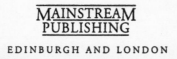

MAINSTREAM
PUBLISHING

EDINBURGH AND LONDON

Copyright © Jan de Vries, 1995
All rights reserved
The moral right of the author has been asserted

First published in Great Britain in 1995 by
MAINSTREAM PUBLISHING COMPANY (EDINBURGH) LTD
7 Albany Street
Edinburgh EH1 3UG

Reprinted 1996

ISBN 1 85158 754 3 (paper)
ISBN 1 85158 755 1 (cloth)

No part of this book may be reproduced or transmitted in any form or
by any means without written permission from the publisher, except by a
reviewer who wishes to quote brief passages in connection with a review
written for insertion in a newspaper, magazine or broadcast

A CIP catalogue record for this book is available from the British Library

Typeset in Perpetua
Printed in Finland by WSOY

Contents

Preface

Some time ago, on a nice summer's day, in the Botanical Gardens in Brisbane, Australia, I was asked a very unusual question during an interview with some Australian journalists. A young journalist asked if I had ever imagined that I might be called upon at some future time to treat royalty and famous people from the theatre and sports world. I had never given the matter much thought, but having been confronted with this question, it made me think back to the scepticism about alternative medicine that was prevalent at the time when I was converted to this form of medicine by Dr Alfred Vogel. In those days we had to battle with the concept that only allopathic medicine could offer acceptable and trustworthy healthcare. Fortunately today, it is with some measure of satisfaction that I see the progress towards a broader spectrum of healthcare and the move towards dispelling some of those narrow-minded beliefs. The question also reminded me just how long ago it was that I first became fascinated by the possibilities of alternative therapies, and I realised that in the year 1995 I had a great deal to celebrate.

I first met Dr Alfred Vogel in 1958, and in 1959 we started working together. It was not until 1960, however, that I was appointed as the first director of what has since grown to be the largest manufacturer of herbal and homoeopathic remedies in the Netherlands. That is now thirty-five years ago and ever since then we have worked very closely together. There is no doubt that Dr Vogel has been a great mentor. So much has happened because, although my career began in the Netherlands, I did not stay there. This year it is exactly twenty-five years since I arrived in Scotland, where I set up a clinic offering treatment with natural medicine on the West coast, in the small town of Troon in Ayrshire. Never in my wildest imagination could I have foreseen that this clinic would grow as it has. Together with my many co-workers we have sometimes treated as many as two thousand patients in one week.

I recently realised that this would be my twenty-fifth book and therefore it has been given twenty-five chapters. Furthermore, in 1995 my wife and I will also celebrate our thirty-fifth wedding anniversary, and we have four daughters who are all, in some way, involved in medicine, either orthodox or alternative.

Although this book is primarily meant to provide practical help for people on a number of different health-related subjects, it might be somewhat anecdotal here and there, where I have drawn upon some of the experiences I have encountered in my seven clinics. I am still very much involved in practices in the Netherlands; in Troon, Scotland; in Belfast, Northern Ireland and in Preston, London and Newcastle in England. Indeed, this wide variety of clinics in contrasting settings and environments results in a great mix of patients and medical conditions.

I sincerely hope that this book will be of help to the many people who, like me thirty-five years ago, are looking for other ways of treating the body that are more in line with the laws of nature, and who wish to be more in tune with nature. After all, it is true what Dr Vogel used to emphasise in most of his lectures: in nature everything is in balance. Man has destroyed much of this balance, but it should never be forgotten that this force of nature will always heal.

1

What is Health?

As one of the oldest universities in Europe, Edinburgh University has had its share of distinguished visitors. The story goes that an important visitor was once asked a question by one of his medical peers: 'What is health?' Because this visitor believed in the laws of opposites his initial response took the form of yet another question: 'What is illness?' He then went on to answer that question by stating that illness is disharmony. This important visitor was no less than the founder of homoeopathy, the German doctor Samuel Hahnemann, who lived from 1755 to 1843. I often wonder if this man, with his controversial beliefs, realised at the time how much impact his ideas would make on the world. With regard to the many new, so-called twentieth-century diseases, we must reconsider Hahnemann's answer when asked for his definition of health. If the definition of illness is disharmony, then it goes without saying that health must be harmony. In the case of illness something has gone wrong in the body; in other words something is out of harmony or out of balance, and in order to find a cure we must first discover the cause.

When I studied in China I gained a better appreciation of what harmony is all about. There I visited the big square in Peking and the Temple of Supremacy. This led to the Temple of Perfection – and can one improve on perfection? According to the Chinese one obviously can, because the Temple of Perfection is followed by the Temple of Harmony. Certainly, illness is disharmony and finding the reason for the disharmony leads us to the main principles laid down by Hahnemann in the laws of homoeopathy. Health depends upon how well we adapt ourselves to internal and external changes. The practitioner plays a secondary role, because he is only the channel. When applying Hahnemann's principles of homoeopathy we must first focus on finding the cause, as it is not the *symptoms* that should be treated, but the *cause* of the disharmony or illness. This makes sense if we think of the analogy that when the church is on fire and the bells are ringing, stopping the pealing of the bells will not put out the fire. If we do not bring out the firehose the fire will not be extinguished. The bells act as an alarm to convey that there is something wrong. So it is with illness. So often people take a tablet to subdue the pain, but this will not touch the root of the problem. The symptoms of pain or discomfort are a warning that somewhere in the body something is wrong – something is out of harmony.

It was this reasoning that attracted me to study drugs. Unfortunately, all too often drugs are prescribed to overcome the symptoms, without consideration for the underlying cause, which therefore remains untreated. Hahnemann insisted on finding and treating the cause of the problem, which in today's terminology makes him a holistic practitioner. When I see people in my clinic with causative factors that have not been treated or removed, I can easily understand why it is sometimes stated that by suppressing disease we are rapidly creating a nation of chronic invalids. Suppression of an illness has no value, because the illness should be brought out and treated.

I remember a young man I saw not so long ago in my clinic in Northern Ireland. He was a tall, pleasant person, who clearly looked unwell. I asked him if he had had glandular fever and he replied that that was how his malaise had started. I told him that as far as I was concerned he was still suffering from glandular fever because his lymph glands were very swollen. He admitted that he often felt feverish and miserable. He had been prescribed antibiotics for his glandular fever, but the illness had obviously never left his system completely. I have often seen that a miasma can remain present for a long time, a miasma being a leftover from a previous inflammation, virus or infection. I started the treatment of this young man by prescribing some homoeopathic remedies to bring out the miasma. When I saw him a while later his condition had already begun to improve.

Even the smallest miasma can lead to major problems. I remember the case of another patient, a girl who came to me with the diagnosis that she was suffering from multiple sclerosis (MS). Before I performed certain tests I asked her if the MS diagnosis was conclusive, and she replied that her doctor had been somewhat doubtful, but could not come up with anything more precise. I told her that I was doubtful that she had MS, although her system was under a great deal of stress and she was unable to walk. When I learned that she took the oral contraceptive pill this was reason enough for me to investigate further. It became apparent that, unfortunately, she was allergic to the pill, a situation I had come across several times before. I prescribed a powerful homoeopathic potency to bring about a healing crisis, and in the middle of the night her fiance phoned to tell me that she was very ill and running a high temperature. I congratulated him and he was taken aback because I did not volunteer to visit her. I told him that I would come and see her the next morning.

I understand that this may appear uncaring to the reader, but I will explain. In his experiments Hahnemann discovered that remedies obtained from animal, vegetable, mineral and biological material could be extremely effective in even the smallest potencies. From this, he arrived at his principle: *'Similia similibus curantur'* – 'Let like be treated by like'. In other words, if you have a cold and sniff a peeled onion, your cold will get worse, but it will leave the system very much sooner. When Hahnemann himself tried the drug cinchona, he was amazed to discover that it produced in him the very symptoms of the disease which it was supposed to cure. When he repeated the experiment, using different drugs with other volunteers, his findings led to a reinforcement of the great healing principle, first pronounced by Paracelsus. In this way Hahnemann paved the way for the future of homoeopathy, which allows for the successful treatment of twentieth-century diseases by selecting a remedy that corresponds to the problem.

The importance of Hahnemann's principle becomes clear when we recognise that in MS patients, a miasma of measles has often been traced, or sometimes an allergy has been discovered in the background. After things had been brought to a head with my young patient the doctor who had diagnosed her as suffering from MS contacted me. By this time she was on the mend and had started to learn to walk again. She had told her doctor about the crisis and he wanted to know more about it. I explained about the homoeopathic potency I had given her, and he complimented me on my diagnosis of detecting the oral contraceptive pill as an allergen. Although not unknown, this is fortunately not a common occurrence. It is, however, possible that a minor factor may have major consequences and therefore it is important to ensure that all factors are considered when diagnosing a patient's ailment. From my conversation with this girl's doctor I realised he was still sceptical and that he doubted that such a small homoeopathic potency could possibly be effective. I know that it is very difficult to prove the effectiveness of homoeopathic remedies, but I have often witnessed that once the homoeopathic potency mixes with the patient's saliva it can affect the person's life force. It may be hard for scientists to understand, but I will quote from an article written in a Dutch newspaper dated 14 November 1994:

It has been scientifically proven that the principle on which homoeopathy has been based is effective. A group of twenty-six students of molecular cell biology at the University of Utrecht have published the results of a four-year research project on animal cells. According to the project leader, human cells are largely identical to animal cells. The conclusion, therefore, is that the principle will be equally effective on human beings.

The research has shown that the cell recovers more quickly if a low potency of the matter that has caused the damage is administered. In homoeopathy this phenomenon is referred to as the 'similia principle'.

The project group initially purposely damaged the cells (with arsenic and cadmium), after which the same matter was administered in very diluted form. The result was that those cells that received the low-potency dilution healed considerably faster than the cells that had to find healing from within themselves. Furthermore, the cells developed an extra resistance to the offensive matter.

According to the research group, it is, however, absolutely essential that the same matter is used in the potency as that which caused the damage in the first place, or else a matter that is very closely related to the offender. It was useless to use an unrelated matter.

The researchers intend to prove their findings with at least two further offensive matters, of which zinc is one. They intend to use a radical system in order to determine whether the principle is equally effective in seriously damaged cells.

This account helps us to understand more clearly why homoeopathic practitioners set so much store on reaching a healing crisis. The research group also found that in order to overcome the original problem it was advantageous to promote a crisis. This is in line with the principles of naturopathy. My grandmother used to say 'Give me influenza and I can treat every ill.' By this she meant that with the help of a bout of influenza it was possible to bring the underlying illness out of the system. By suppressing a disease we compound the problem, and this becomes more evident with the so-called twentieth-century diseases such as myalgic encephalomyelitis (ME), allergies and auto-immune diseases. It is my experience that these diseases are often the result of an underlying illness having been suppressed. We should work towards this crisis and I have often seen that the illness must travel back the same road from which it came. Sometimes patients phone me in distress because their condition has worsened; even though I have warned them beforehand of this possibility, in their anxiety they seem to forget this. When such a crisis approaches, there is frequently an increase in body temperature, but this is desirable in bringing the illness or condition to its conclusion. This generally happens with illnesses such as ME, which is often thought to be the result of a suppressed illness, similarly with *Candida albicans*, a condition which can be caused by taking too many antibiotics. This explains why there is no cause for undue worry when a healing crisis occurs, as long as we look at the body holistically.

The phrase 'holistic medicine' is often used in the USA and is based on Hahnemann's principles of treating mind, body and soul. In lectures I often explain that man has three bodies: a physical body, a mental body and an emotional body. These three bodies should be in harmony, and if one of these bodies is out of harmony the individual's overall wellbeing is affected.

All too often I see that treatment is specifically directed towards problems in the physical body, ignoring the possibility of the illness originating in the mental or emotional body. This insular outlook became very clear during my involvement in a four-year research project on arthritis and rheumatism. The inflammatory conditions were being attacked by strong drugs, sometimes aggressively, to try and control the inflammation. Arthritis and rheumatism are thought to be most commonly caused by infections, allergies or inherited weaknesses. I saw that many of those patients had problems in their emotional or mental body: tensions resulting from unemployment, jealousy, marital problems, etc. If we take into consideration the mental and emotional problems and observe the three bodies of the patient, we might be more successful in our treatments. I often feel that this is where medicine, in its totality, has failed. I concede that, initially, a rheumatologist, by sometimes attacking those problems aggressively, may achieve a speedier result than I could. From experience with my patients, however, by treating the three bodies of man, the longer-term results are better. So often physical problems can be triggered by an emotional upset. Such problems can develop from relatively minor disharmonies, going on to disturb not only the physical body, but also the mental and emotional bodies. Therefore the term 'holistic medicine' more accurately describes the necessary approach.

While I was preparing to write about this subject I remembered a case history from quite a number of years ago. It concerned a girl who was brought to me when I was lecturing in Canada. She was extremely ill and I was told that if I was wearing after-shave I should not approach her because it was likely to make her faint. The various doctors who had examined this girl could not agree on a diagnosis. ME had been mentioned, and so had hyperventilation and hyperallergy. I discussed her case with a few of my Canadian colleagues and with our combined forces we successfully tackled the problem. I remained in close contact with the girl's parents, who kept me informed of her progress. When we first saw this girl her condition was very poor indeed. Eventually, we learned that this poor girl had been raped when she was very young. This sad situation had affected her emotional body like a poison, and had subsequently involved the mental and physical bodies so that her system had become very toxic, as if it was truly being poisoned. This is not unusual, because we are well aware that emotions, anxieties and stress very often lead to a toxic body. There was much work to be done. I cannot tell you how happy I was when, during my most recent visit to Canada for a lecture tour, she offered to join me on the platform and tell the audience her life story. She had fully recovered and had also regained her confidence, and was prepared to share her experiences in an effort to help others.

This story provides us with an excellent example of why treatment of these three bodies should take place simultaneously, and this is one of the major principles of homoeopathy. It is unfortunate that homoeopathy is sometimes unfairly attacked as a religion, because it has nothing whatsoever to do with religion. Homoeopathy is a *scientific* approach, the usefulness of which has once again been confirmed by the research findings I quoted earlier. Success depends largely on the practitioner choosing the correct remedy for the individual. Constitutional remedies are very important in homoeopathy. The appropriate dosage of the right remedy must be prescribed and for this too, the practitioner's experience is very important. Complex remedies sometimes work in a different manner, but the fact remains that one simple remedy can cause a minor vibration capable of causing a change in a patient's condition. It was Isaac Newton who said, 'When one atom vibrates, the whole universe is shaken.'

Hahnemann was also intent on preserving the good in his aim to stamp out the bad. We see too often that the body is aggressively bombarded with chemicals or drugs in an attempt to destroy diseased cells, but at the same time these therapies also destroy healthy cells. This is often the case with antibiotics. The discovery of antibiotics was a major breakthrough in medicine and has proved to be a blessing to mankind. Sir Alexander Fleming, who lived not very far from our clinic in the West of Scotland, discovered penicillin. I know his family and I have tremendous respect for his discovery. However, Alexander Fleming never intended for antibiotics to be prescribed and taken like sweets, but unfortunately this appears to be a common occurrence nowadays. The word *antibiotics* in fact means *anti-life*:they are a means of destroying what is bad, but unfortunately also kill the good at the same time. The increase in candida problems, is largely due to excessive use of antibiotics. Of course, antibiotics can be a great salvation, but they should be used in the full knowledge of what they actually do.

On one occasion I accepted an invitation to give a lecture to several hundred doctors in Germany. I was asked to speak on the effect of viruses and allergies on the immune system. I had a very interested audience and this became particularly clear during question time. This is a slot I usually schedule at the end of my lectures. One of the less scientific questions was directed at finding out what my secret was because I had been asked to treat so many famous people. I told those present that I had no secrets and that I was prepared to share any knowledge, as I had done in the lecture that had just finished. During this lecture I had spoken about a number of remedies on which I was very dependent for the treatment of my patients. I reminded them that I had mentioned *Echinacea purpurea*, or Echinaforce. Without this remedy I would not have been able to help half the people I have treated, and therefore I often refer to it as my best friend and ally. It has never failed me and in cases where an antibiotic was necessary, or in the case of a penicillin allergy or immunity, Echinaforce has been essential. I reminded them that I had already explained the characteristics of the plant *Echinacea* and pointed out that the strength and immunity of that plant and flower is confirmed by the fact that the *Echinacea* plant will not wither if it does not receive any water, even if it is kept dry for a considerable period of time. Moreover, these characteristics are maintained when this plant is used in the preparation of remedies. In many cases it has proved itself to be more powerful than any chemical compound antibiotic.

I noticed some disbelief among my audience and some of them were openly critical. However, I received unexpected, but tremendous support from one of the doctors present, who spoke out in my defence. She asked if she could be allowed to tell us about a personal experience. She told the gathering that when she had been travelling in Brazil, she had developed an abscess in the mouth and she could not find a chemist to purchase any antibiotics. Finally, she found a little healthfood store and, remembering that her grandmother had always recommended chamomile, she explained her predicament to the owner. She was correct, because for oral infections a gargle with a chamomile infusion, as hot as possible, may render the offending bacteria harmless. The owner of the healthfood store did not have any chamomile, but he recommended Echinaforce without hesitation in the circumstances. He only had one bottle left on the shelf, but it was hers if she wanted it. She read the recommended dosage on the label –

three times daily, fifteen drops before meals – and decided to double the dose. This lady happily told my audience that day in Germany that the abscess had burst that very same evening after she had taken a double dose three times over the course of the day. The next day she felt marvellous again. This is the kind of audience participation no public speaker can object to. This story also shows that strong remedies, which destroy the good along with the bad and are likely to cause side-effects elsewhere in the body, are not always necessary.

Then there is Hahnemann's respect for the life force in the body. This life force is so incredibly strong that it is often under-estimated. Yet, in our daily lives this life force is under constant attack from the pollution of our food, water and air – three life-giving substances without which life would not be possible. This life force is essential for maintaining good health. Where circumstances cause a minor erosion, harmony will be destroyed. Anything that attacks this life force will affect our energy and our immune system. We can maintain our good health if we positively work at keeping this life force strong within us. A good, wholesome diet and natural remedies will help and this was one of the first things that attracted me to Dr Vogel's philosophies. From him I learned to regard the body in its entirety and I also found that he was one of the few people who saw a plant, herb or a flower in the same way. In his remedies he uses the whole plant and obtains an extract by a carefully controlled process. I remember the many times we would take a walk in the Swiss Alps, when he would point to a plant and explain what its characteristics were. It was Dr Vogel who taught me that by looking at a plant it is often possible to identify a disease or illness for which this plant may be useful. In Creation everything is in balance and only if we find harmony in these three bodies of man can we find an answer to the question of what health is all about.

I have now been involved in the world of alternative medicine for thirty-five years, but I will never forget the first day I met Dr Vogel and how, as a result of his teachings, my future changed radically. In today's society the value of these teachings becomes clearer when we wonder, or ask ourselves, what is to become of the human race.

2

A Healthy Heart

'Keep the heart with all diligence for out of it are the issues of life.' These words appear in Proverbs 4:24; they were written by King Solomon and I sometimes wonder if he had been influenced by his father, the great King David, when he wrote them. My reason for saying this is that King David often spoke of the heart, the kidneys and the mind being tested by our Creator. In fact, all through the Bible we find that certain parts of the body are mentioned as providing pointers towards an understanding of the three bodies – the physical, mental and emotional bodies – of man.

I remember that during my studies one of my professors would frequently remind us that the mind is a mental state, the heart is an emotional state, the soul is a spiritual state and the body is a physical state, and that a harmonious relationship between these bodies is necessary for good health.

Sometimes I used to stay overnight with some friends when I attended my clinic in the Midlands in England, and I remember a particularly interesting conversation we had one evening. We discussed the stresses of life at a time when my friends were going through a particularly difficult period themselves. It was a very stimulating evening, and we had all been very honest with ourselves and each other. We certainly had food for thought when we retired. At about two o'clock in the morning the lady of the house knocked on my bedroom door to ask for help because her husband was not at all well. I went to see him immediately and he was indeed very distressed. I was about to call for an ambulance when he seemed to settle. We eventually went back to bed, but I had to insist that he should see his own doctor the next day, because his heart was under tremendous strain and causing him great discomfort.

The heart is often an indicator of a person's emotional state. The stresses and tensions of life affect the heart to such an extent that it sometimes can give us a fright, as it did with my friend. Fortunately, because I was there to help him that night, he is still very much alive and active, even though he should have retired some time ago. The action I took that night was to give him some Cardiaforce, and after a little while I also gave him some Crataegisan, a remedy derived from the hawthorn berry. Although I have worked with these remedies for many years, I am still amazed how obvious the signatures and characteristics of nature are. The hawthorn berry has been used for remedial purposes by many previous generations and that red berry is reminiscent of the heart, which is the motor of life. The heart is such an enormously important part of our life that we should diligently care for it. When the heart is calm and not overstressed this is reflected in the whole of the body. Again I quote King Solomon, who said that 'a sound heart is the life of the flesh'. If we think of the heart in a holistic context, it is not surprising that it is affected by any illness or disease.

I remember a young patient, whom I had known for a number of years as a carefree girl, and a happy young woman. Unfortunately, when she came to see me it was because she had experienced great emotional problems. She had been very much in love with her boyfriend, and when he eventually dropped her she had not been able accept this. I realised that I was looking at someone who was dying of a broken heart. Emotionally, the heart is easily affected. Indeed, it would be wrong to regard the heart as no more than a physical organ.

From the physical aspect, however, we must marvel at the tremendous job the heart performs. I have practised for many years in Scotland, and it has saddened me to learn that Scotland supposedly has the highest mortality rate in the world due to heart disease. Yet this problem extends throughout the industrialised world. The official figures for Australia estimate that approximately 50,000 people die of cardio-vascular disease every year, which is approximately 1,000 people every week. The statistics are certainly not much better in countries like the USA and the UK.

You will appreciate that the heart must be a very strong muscular pump, because its weight is only approximately 10oz. To sustain life the heart has to beat about forty million times a year and it supplies every organ and all the tissue in the body with blood. The heart is a beautifully designed mechanism and in simple terms it functions as follows: the heart muscle contracts and pumps our blood, and the blood vessels and coronary arteries carry oxygen and nourishment to the heart muscle and the valves, through which the blood enters and leaves the heart. These very important parts constitute the task and function of the heart. It is essential that the heart muscle also receives enough oxygen to supply the small arteries, some of which are only one-eighth of an inch in diameter. A well-functioning aortic valve is of the greatest importance.

Sometimes we are guilty of not paying enough attention to our health, and this will catch up with us sooner or later. This happened to one of my old friends, a well-known and successful artist who spent his life fulfilling one commission after the other, without considering his health. He later admitted that he should have paid attention to some of the early warning signs. When he did eventually go for a medical check-up he was told that it was essential to undergo immediate surgery in order to avoid major complications.

I certainly don't want to encourage people to become hypochondriacs or neurotics – there is already an abundance of them. Nevertheless, I must stress that the messages given out by the body should not be ignored. Pay attention if you suddenly become aware of unusual tiredness, or if you notice that your heart rate is irregular, whether it be slower or faster. The body is so well designed that it will emit alarm signals, relaying the message that something is not functioning properly. Seek treatment before bigger problems arise.

Now let's look at what really happens when someone has a heart attack. First we will look at the coronary arteries, those vital blood vessels that transport the blood to the heart muscle itself. In babies and young children the inner lining of the coronary arteries is smooth and flexible, and the arteries are supple and elastic. The coronary arteries connect with the ventricles, receiving and pumping blood to the chambers of the heart. Artery branches extend over the surface of the heart, and the heart supplies these arteries with oxygen, mixed with carbon dioxide and other waste nutrients. However, with advancing age, or possibly because of poor physical care, problems can arise. The artery lining becomes gradually discoloured and thickens, and there is a deposit of fatty material. Then there can be danger. Problems like intermittent claudication, or the arteries to the brain being affected, or blood vessels bursting and causing haemorrhages can occur, and therefore it is important that we learn how these can be avoided.

Maintaining the correct blood pressure is very important in this process and in order to understand how coronary disease can be avoided, we should know what the important factors are:

1. the strength of the heart
2. the volume of blood sent out from the heart
3. resistance in the capillaries, especially those in the kidneys
4. the resilience of the artery walls
5. the tone of the vegetative nerve network

6. the delicate responses in the parasympathetic and the sympathetic nerve balance.

The *diastolic*, or tissue, pressure equals the resistance to the flow of blood in the tissues and the *systolic* pressure equals the diastolic pressure plus pulse pressure. Systolic pressure occurs as the heart cavities contract and force blood onwards, and diastolic pressure as the heart cavities expand and fill with blood. Again, one affects the other, and there are four million reflexes to the heart which act to raise or lower systolic blood pressure. From the point of view of an acupuncture therapist, the heart reflex in the foot slows the heart and makes it beat stronger. The reflexes in the left hand and in the arm above the elbow, make the heart beat regularly. Near the left eye is another reflex that makes heart beat faster and stronger. To raise and lower the diastolic pressure, reflexes to the kidneys, adrenals and the rectum are used. These are found in the foot and head zones. Many people know that a pain in the inner side of the left arm is usually indicative of some disorder of the coronary arteries. Always bear in mind that the digestive system, from the mouth to the anus, is most important, and in acupuncture I always treat these points.

It is possible to do this by treating the lymphatics and the kidneys, or even through the feet and hands, by balancing these predestined zones. Unfortunately, the lymphatics rarely receive the attention they warrant.

The digestive system plays a remarkably important role in heart disease and the feared expression 'Eat yourself to a diseased heart' is often proved to be correct. I once attended a Rotary dinner as an invited guest and while we were all conversing and enjoying ourselves, I noticed a friend of mine across the table turning very pale and then suddenly he slumped and fell off his chair. Fortunately, we were able to give him first aid, but he had suffered a severe heart attack, probably brought on by the momentary over-eating and over-drinking, with which his digestive system was unable to cope. I always emphasise to heart patients that they should watch their weight, masticate their food very thoroughly and to keep their meals small and simple. Large and rich meals can take their toll.

Tension is, of course, another important factor, and nowadays there is so much fear, stress and tension in our lives that the incidence of coronary thrombosis and other heart conditions is ever increasing.

It was in 1912 that a heart attack was first medically recognised, but it was not until 1925 that medicine began to gain some understanding of this problem. Why should it be that we now see such a tremendous increase in heart problems? There are a number of relevant factors: fear, worry, and tension are widely recognised as contributory factors, but the enormous change in diet is also a major influence. Before the 1930s the rich had a completely different diet to the poor, but nowadays the food intake for both rich and poor is excessive – too much sugar, salt and fat, as well as too much stress. I always say that our major enemies can be summed up in the three S's, i.e. salt, sugar and stress. These results of a higher standard of living have had a detrimental effect on our health. It is sometimes said that we kill our loved ones with kindness, and this is not far from the truth. It may be interesting to know that during the Second World War there was a much lower incidence of heart disease and stomach and bowel problems. The little there was to eat in occupied countries was largely roughage, and although that by no means constituted a healthy diet, and there was widespread evidence of malnutrition, standards of general health were higher than today.

In my book *Heart and Blood Circulatory Problems* I have repeatedly stated that cholesterol is a major enemy of our health. This substance, if it settles as a jellied mass on the inner wall of the arteries, can cause them to clog. However, it is more significant that those little particles that travel through the arteries, where they sometimes settle, are mostly caused by excessive intake of animal fats, alcohol and nicotine. Also, few people take sufficient exercise, and instead of using our legs to get the messages from the corner shop, we are in the habit of taking the car – using our legs as extensions of the car pedals. This may be a novel idea, but it is not doing us any good. Walking is such an exhilarating and healthy form of exercise. I remember reading an article about an athlete who went running for at least one hour every day. At his death at the age of sixty-nine a post mortem was performed, and it was remarkable how healthy his heart was. Doctors pronounced that his heart was in the same condition as might be expected of a male in his early twenties. I am sure that it was totally different with King Henry VIII, who was renowned for eating enormous meals every day and whose health suffered badly because of it. Today, lots of people live like that king of the realm, only storing fat for the future, to the detriment of their health. There is a great deal of truth in the saying that you are what you eat, and therefore it is important to keep the heart in good condition, because the heart is the motor for our body. Protect against stress and take sufficient exercise, and together these precautions will undoubtedly result in a stronger heart.

Of the numerous cases I have been asked to treat during my many years in practice those that especially sadden me are congenital and inherited conditions. We know that the embryo's heart develops during the first ten weeks of pregnancy, and that approximately one in every three hundred babies born is a so-called 'blue baby', in other words a baby with a congenital heart condition. Sadly, some of these babies die in their infancy, depending on the severity of the deformity. At other times, thanks to the remarkable modern medical techniques, developed especially during the last decade, these young children can be given corrective surgery enabling them to survive and subsequently lead a full life.

The various heart conditions each require a different approach, but in general terms wonderful remedies such as Arnica, Crataegus, *Spigaelia*, and even *Avena sativa*, can sometimes be helpful. If there is a problem with body fluids a homoeopathic potency of lily of the valley can be helpful, even if the patient is on long-term medication prescribed by his or her specialist. It is believed that this flower has been used for medicinal purposes for at least four hundred years, yet many of us have this flower growing in our own garden without appreciating its medicinal characteristics. This flower has also been called 'Return of Happiness' and, possibly because of its pure white colour and its sweet fragrance, it was believed to have the power of pointing mankind in the direction of a better life. This explains why, even in modern times, a bridal bouquet often contains a sprig of lily of the valley.

Happiness is of the greatest importance in terms of our health, and especially so for a heart patient. Rarely a day goes past without me being reminded of the three bodies: physical, mental and emotional. Last week I again saw a patient who had probably one of the most serious heart conditions I have ever treated. When I first saw him some three or four years ago, his blood pressure was shockingly high. His heart was in an extremely poor condition and his prospects looked grim, and with all that he still had to keep a demanding and thriving business going. His wife was very caring and supportive and told me how worried she was about him. Fortunately, his doctor was kind enough to send me details of his condition. As well as the weakness in his heart he had angina pectorus. Certainly, this man was in desperate need of help. It was absolutely essential that he changed his dietary habits and, fortunately, he was aware of the seriousness of his condition and so decided to follow my advice to the letter.

I prescribed some remedies that would help to strengthen his heart and to control his angina. First of all we set about lowering his cholesterol level, in which we were soon successful, and he began to show a slight general improvement. However, about a year ago I learned that his wife had died. I was extremely concerned, as was his general practitioner. Fortunately, he has come through this emotionally stressful period, but neither his own practitioner nor I have found a real cure. To some extent he did that himself when he found a new wife, filling his life with happiness. I am sure that body chemistries have done something for him: when I saw him last week his blood pressure was fine and so was his heart rhythm, he was glowing with happiness and I was strengthened in my belief that the third body – the emotional body – is of vital importance to our general health. This man's physical condition cannot be cured, but he is managing to control it better and it is this new-found happiness that has enabled him to do so. The improvement in his angina condition has been so remarkable that it prompted his specialist to enquire what he had done. He told him that first of all he had given up smoking and drinking, he had reduced his intake of coffee and tea, watched his diet, and that he was taking some homoeopathic remedies. One of the finest remedies for him was *Viscum album* (extract of mistletoe), together with Hyperisan, which is derived from *Hypericum perforatum*. As he had many problems with constipation, he also used a quarter teaspoon of Linoforce twice a day, which ensures a regular bowel function. Hence his great dietary efforts saved the day.

It is amazing how many people have an irregular heartbeat, and they will often benefit from the homoeopathic remedy wolf's claw, or *Lycopus europaeus*. A few drops of this remedy will generally calm and reduce a rapid heartbeat, which seems to be more common in young people, who are particularly concerned by such symptoms. In general, I may recommend the remedy Kelpasan, possibly with some Urticalcin, or a supplementary vitamin preparation such as Imuno-Strength or Health Insurance Plus. Co-Enzyme Q10 has also proved very useful and I would certainly recommend three garlic capsules to be taken at night.

I have reached that age in my life when I more frequently receive news of the death of one of my contemporaries or of one of my friends. In many cases I learn that this death has been due to a heart attack and I know that the stress and tensions of life have claimed yet another victim. I remember being worried about my own health a few years ago, and I went for help to a friend whom I have known since our days at university. He gave me a thorough check-over and assured me that everything was all right, but added that I had a 'sport heart' at that time. I knew that this was possibly my own fault because I was working very long hours and because of my great energy I sometimes have to stop myself and make sure that I get enough rest and relaxation. Prevention is better than cure.

Many heart problems result from disharmony in other body organs or functions, but in all cases it is important to pay attention to diet and to be

23

prepared to make changes. A healthy diet lowers the cholesterol level. Stop smoking and keep alcohol to the minimum. Take regular exercise and learn to relax. Have your blood pressure checked at regular intervals. Remember the three 'S's' – salt, sugar and stress – and make sure you have an adequate intake of fibre in your diet to ensure a good bowel function. Fat is another problem that should be watched carefully and by this I mean the kind of fat that is eaten. All diets need to contain fat, but do make sure that they are of the right type, such as polyunsaturated or essential fats. Saturated fats have no dietary value and these are found in beef, pork, lamb, lard, hard margarines, dairy products, cakes, biscuits and pastries. When eating meat, cut off the fat, because then the diet will be less harmful, and although poultry tends to be less fatty, here also it should be borne in mind that any fat should be discarded. Fish is much more advisable. If you cannot bear to cut out salt, please try and reduce your intake, and consider replacing it with sea salt, or one of the excellent substitutes such as Dr Vogel's Herbamare or Trocamare. Instead of sugar you may like to consider using honey. Coffee substitutes or herbal teas are much better than the usual beverages. Eat plenty of fruit and vegetables, especially apples, garlic, onions, aubergines, beans and soya. All this is simple advice, but it will be rewarding.

As far as supplements are concerned, it is wise to take some extra vitamins, minerals and trace elements and I often advise the use of Herbal Health Complex to try and keep the heart healthy. This is a herbal combination that includes vitamins, minerals and trace elements. This remedy has proved successful as a preventive measure, especially in cases of arteriosclerosis.

Perfect health is a very difficult term to define, because every human being is born with some cells of degeneration or some inherited problem. I am impressed with the definition of the World Health Organisation (WHO): 'Health is a state of complete physical, mental and social well-being, and not merely the absence of disease or infirmity.' Many supplements that are beneficial to general health are also of value for those with heart conditions, for example vitamin C, vitamin E and Oil of Evening Primrose.

During question time after a recent lecture to the medical staff in a hospital, I mentioned Oil of Evening Primrose. When I explained how necessary this substance is as it provides an essential fatty acid which is so often lacking in the diet nowadays, one of the students protested that I placed too much emphasis on this nutritional supplement. I then told the gathering that I was one of the first practitioners to prescribe Oil of

Evening Primrose capsules in Great Britain and because of my long experience I had great faith in this supplement. The student denied that it could possibly be of such great value and suggested it was only yet another ploy to line the manufacturer's pockets. As he was Scottish I asked him if he was familiar with the work of Robert Burns, the well-known Scottish poet, and although surprised, he agreed that he very much appreciated his poetry and could recite long sections of it by heart. I then explained to him that Robert Burns once wrote in a letter to his friend Dr Moore that 'the blunders and the mistakes we make today is often to our ignorance'. This student took offence and asked whether I considered him ignorant. I explained that although Oil of Evening Primrose was ridiculed when I started prescribing it some thirty years ago, it is now prescribed by many doctors and is even available on prescription. He admitted that he had not been aware of this and he was quite taken aback. I quote here from a poem written in the eighteenth century:

> Life unseen by moonlight glow, lovely flower unseen;
> your seeds will restore the vital power . . .

This quote is thought to refer to the evening primrose, and I would not be surprised if its medicinal characteristics were known even then. The heart muscle will certainly be strengthened with the use of vitamin E and Oil of Evening Primrose. Vitamin B complex will particularly restore the nerve tension of the heart. Vitamin C will help to build healthy walls for the veins and arteries, and garlic capsules will keep the arteries supple and flexible.

In the case of serious heart problems oral chelation therapy is of tremendous value. A healthy artery can easily develop some fatty streaks, something we are rarely aware of in the early stages. This is usually followed by plaque, which can cause thrombosis, or calcification, possibly resulting in a haemorrhage. Oral chelation therapy is advantageous in avoiding or arresting the development of such problems and I have seen some very encouraging results when my patients have used products such as Oral Nutrient Chelate, or Oral Chelate.

The liver also plays a significant role in maintaining a healthy heart because it breaks down lipids, which are fatty substances, and keeps cholesterol soluble so that it can be excreted. Lipotropid factors, such as betasitosterol methionine and betaine, support the healthy flow of fat and bile. Proper calcium absorption is also important. When the body fluids become overly alkaline, calcium can be thrown out of solution.

Magnesium and potassium are widely recognised for their role in maintaining the condition of the heart muscle and its force of concentration. Oral chelation formulas provide these vital nutrients together with synergistic factors and these formulas are often of great value.

The heart is also an emotional state. Physically, there are many ways that we can help it, but emotionally, with the help of your loved ones, there is much you can do yourself to improve your condition. We are all familiar with expressions such as 'a broken heart', 'the heart beating in the mouth', 'a heart of gold', or even 'a heart of stone'. Such phrases are widely used to indicate one's emotional condition, but they do not describe a physical phenomenon. Such emotional conditions, however, do express themselves in physical disorders. If you have read my book *Body Energy* you will know that I advise that we listen to the language of our body. Do not ignore the messages emitted by the body that indicate that something is out of sorts. For example, the expression 'I have a heavy heart' is commonly used after some unusual exertion, either mental or physical. This is a warning that we are taking on responsibilities that are too great. I always remember my mother's advice that one should have a brief moment of contemplation before going to sleep. Look into your heart and ask yourself if your day was well spent: have I done the right thing; have I been honest; have I been loving enough to those around me; have I done my daily duties; have I been an example to others and am I in harmony with God and nature?

3

A Healthy Liver

I used to wonder why Dr Vogel gave his book *The Liver* the subtitle *The Regulator of Health*, but over the years I have come to understand the meaning of that message only too well. The book's subtitle becomes self-explanatory in the light of some of the case histories where the liver was affected. Some time ago, a rabbi and his wife made an appointment at my clinic. He came into the consulting room arguing with his wife and he was taken aback when I asked him about his liver problems. He asked if I had second sight, but I explained that by looking at him I could tell that he had a liver condition. When he agreed that this was the case I advised him that the best thing to do was to stop arguing with his wife. Their relationship was a big problem for both of them. They irritated each other immensely because both of them were argumentative and the result was that he became very wound up. I got the impression that they were not well suited, and quite possibly this was the cause of his ill health. The rabbi's wife told me that every time her husband had a liver upset she had to suffer the sharp edge of his tongue, whereupon I told the rabbi that in his position, where he should be an example to others, he could not afford to be like that. If he changed his attitude he would probably be a more contented and pleasant person. He has taken my words to heart and has indeed become a much happier person.

This rabbi was like King Henry VIII in that he ate and drank whatever and whenever he felt like it, so placing unrealistic demands on his liver. When his physical condition upset him, his poor wife had to bear the brunt of it. I firmly believe that emotional stress takes its toll on the physical body. It has sometimes been disputed by colleagues when I say that in serious cases of nervous tension the liver is always affected. I have seen it with patients who were unwilling to give up alcohol or cigars, until eventually they have been forced to do so because their liver could not cope with the abuse. I have seen so many unhappy marriages where the husband or wife took to drink or drugs, until finally the liver has called a halt. Therefore I have come to believe, like Dr Vogel, that the liver is indeed the regulator of health.

The liver is greatly influenced by what we eat and drink and this is because nutrition is the foundation of health. The digestive process starts when food and drink pass through the mouth, the stomach and the duodenum, and is dependent on amino acids, glucose and essential fatty acids. The absorption process comes into play at the division of nutrients in the small and large intestines. If all is well, the waste matter leaves the body when the nutrients have completed their task, during what is called the elimination process. This entire process influences the blood circulation, which immediately affects the liver. If the blood carries too many toxins, or waste material, the liver cannot do its wonderful job.

The liver is the equivalent of a full-time laboratory which filters 1,200 pints of blood in twenty-four hours, and with this knowledge you will understand what a marvellous function it performs. It is responsible for the delivery of quality blood to the heart, which in turn provides all the other organs with nutrients. The quality of the blood depends on amino acids, glucose, essential fatty acids, enzymes, vitamins, minerals and oxygen, and is responsible for the manufacture and renewal of cells. With every tick of the clock some ten thousand cells die and therefore we are dependent on constant cell renewal.

The liver is not only the regulator of health, it is the regulator of life. Until well into the nineteenth century there was limited scientific medical knowledge, but we now know that life is all about the renewal of cells and cell tissue. This process depends on how well the internal organs work, how we feed them and how we look after them. A good cell renewal process also requires harmony between the three bodies, i.e. the physical, mental and emotional bodies. This harmony can be influenced greatly by what we eat and drink, our mental state and how our emotions are controlled. The liver is an organ with many functions, such as the storage of energy, providing glycogen and influencing the assimilation of carbohydrates, amino acids, glucose, fats and proteins. It has a tremendous task to do, yet we often seem to put every imaginable obstacle in its way with alcohol or nicotine abuse, or poor dietary management. The liver purifies and detoxifies the system and at the slightest hitch the body will give us an alarm signal that the liver cannot cope. Even a small disturbance in liver function can lead to jaundice.

The liver is also a major supplier of energy. When parents tell me that their children appear to be constantly tired I can only guess at how much their liver has to cope with. I find it very disturbing to see young people in particular indulging in alcohol abuse, and it does not surprise me that there are so many cases of hepatitis A, B and even C, attacking the immune system, lowering the energy, and causing vulnerabilty to any infections or invaders.

When I practise at my London clinic I purposely always book in at a YMCA hotel. I like staying there because of the number of young people I meet there. The other day I remarked to my assistant that I felt hopeful for the future when I observed a group of pleasant and well-behaved young people and I noticed that they were sensible in their choice of menu. Sometimes when I am returning from a long day in the clinic I see groups of inebriated young people and I pity them because they never stop to consider the damage they are inflicting on their liver. It is sad because there is not even any point in reasoning with them when they are under the influence of alcohol or drugs. Sometimes they look thin and emaciated and it does not require much imagination to realise that the liver – the supplier of energy – is no longer able to perform that function.

The liver is closely involved in the cell renewal process, which requires amino acids as building blocks, and protein, to build a healthy life. The balance between carbohydrates and protein is easily disturbed by highly addictive carbohydrates. Last year I lost a good friend, who was only forty years old and who had a healthy business and a fantastic future. When I saw him at the clinic he told me that he knew he was drinking too much, but he felt that he needed it. At the same time he wondered if he had cirrhosis of the liver. When the results of his tests came back we were sorry to see that the condition had got a firm grip and, belatedly, he tried to change his diet to include more protein, thinking that he might yet undo the results of his long-standing alcohol addiction. It was too late because the damage was irreversible and the cell degeneration was beyond repair. When we said our farewells I felt sorry for his wife and his promising teenage daughters, and I was determined that it would be my mission to continue warning people about the possible outcome of dietary or nutritional abuse or mismanagement. In such circumstances the ending of a life is even more sad as it need never have taken place.

The liver – a living laboratory – was even in ancient times seen as the 'kernel of life'. Modern science has confirmed that the vital chemical processes which take place in the liver certainly influence the three bodies of man. This wonderful laboratory, which weighs no more than 3 oz has been assigned such a wonderful task that without this organ life cannot be sustained. The liver has a tremendous regenerative potential and it is remarkable how even only a small part can be seen to regenerate itself quickly. However, in the case of cancer, any liver involvement will mean a major health problem.

A great number of vessels are involved in the transport of nutrients and blood to and from the liver. This makes a fascinating picture under the microscope, showing the liver in remarkable detail, with its numerous cells, lobes, lobules and tissue strings. In as short a period as one minute the liver receives and processes about two pints of blood.

The reason Dr Vogel calls the liver the regulator of health is its strategic position with regard to the stomach and bowel industry. Vitamins, minerals and trace elements play an important role and are the building blocks for haemoglobin and for the storage of iron. The liver is highly sensitive to toxins, which in high concentrations can cause great damage to the body, and therefore detoxification is important. The liver also plays a major role in the protein and carbohydrate metabolism, and it has a close relationship with the gall bladder. We should always be careful not to overburden this living laboratory that is home to some 350,000 cells containing one million lobules.

Artificial fertilisers, herbicides, insecticides, pesticides and fungicides will all leave their mark on the liver. The presence of toxins is a sure sign that things are not well and that there is some deep-rooted problem. I always feel happy when I see the outcome in patients who have followed a detoxification programme, such as the Rasayana Course devised by Dr Vogel, because it is such an excellent way to cleanse the liver. We also refer to this course as the Spring Cleansing Course; in addition to eliminating toxins, it improves the bowel action so that the liver does not become overburdened. Many of my patients have also been greatly helped by chewing a few seeds of Linoforce several times a day. This too promotes regular bowel movements and alleviates the task of the liver.

At times I have heard Dr Vogel tell his audience how good it would be to undress and lie out in the garden, with the body covered with rhubarb leaves. He used to say that it was like a herbal ablution and, having lain under these rhubarb leaves for a few hours, one would experience a marvellous sense of well-being afterwards. Hot water applications or hot poultices made with thyme or eucalyptus and applied daily produce excellent results and help the liver as well as the pancreas. Papayaforce and Molkosan are other natural remedies that can be of great help.

Together with Dr Vogel, I designed a special liver diet that has proved to be beneficial to people with a liver condition. This is essentially a fat-free diet, because saturated fats can be very harmful, as are high-protein foods, such as meat, especially anything from the pig. The main points of this diet are outlined below.

Liver Diet

• Take only vegetables, preferably raw. Salads mixed with Molkosan, buttermilk, yoghurt (low-fat). Toasted wholemeal bread, potatoes, Ryvita, sunflower or olive oil, honey. Herbal tea, apple juice, blackcurrant juice. Natural brown rice, grapefruit, grapes and berries.

• Absolutely no coffee, tea, white sugar, white flour (nor products in which these ingredients are used), vinegar, tinned products, meat, fish, butter, fried foods, spices, cucumber, cabbage, cauliflower or spinach. No sweets or chocolates.

• Eat two plates of grated carrots daily. Walk 1–1½ hours. One day in the week hold a fasting day. During that day take only apple juice, chamomile tea and some carrot juice. Twice each day spend fifteen minutes doing breathing exercises.

• *To prepare whole brown rice:* Preheat the oven to a high temperature. Place the rice in a casserole or Pyrex dish and pour over some boiling milk or water. Cook the rice for 10–15 minutes only before switching off the oven. Leave in the oven for 5–6 hours. Chop some vegetables and herbs such as parsley, chicory, celery and cress and mix these through the rice with a little garlic salt. Reheat before serving.

These dietary guidelines will be of excellent help for people with liver problems. In general, fruits, vegetables and nuts are to be recommended, especially artichokes.

Boldocynara, which is primarily based on artichokes, is an extremely useful combination remedy that can sometimes produce remarkable results with people who suffer from liver problems. This remedy has proved to be particularly helpful when a liver patient is also prone to obesity or constipation. This is also the case for liver conditions combined with skin problems or migraines. People with liver conditions are often emotionally very upset, especially if liver cancer has been diagnosed. Yet nature so often surprises us: remember that it will never do to give up hope, because with a positive outlook and a strong will to get better, cancer of the liver need not always be considered as incurable. The necessary healing factors are a correctly balanced diet, deep-breathing exercises, natural remedies, and sometimes also water treatments, such as hot showers or hydrotherapy. Details about a large number of water treatment methods can be found in my book *Water – Healer or Poison?*.

A liver patient, whatever the problem may be, will usually benefit from a holiday by the sea. Other good advice is to drink mineral water, or herbal teas such as chamomile, thyme or milk thistle tea. Homoeopathic remedies such as *Podophyllum peltatum 4x*, *Natrium sulphuricum 6x* or *Argentum nitricum 6x* are often successfully prescribed. People living in big cities are more susceptible to liver conditions because of the lack of oxygen, due to heavy traffic with its resultant emissions into the atmosphere. Walking and breathing in the fresh air will give the liver a treat, whereas the skins of people with a sedentary lifestyle, who smoke and drink, will eventually display signs that their liver is being pushed to the limit. I would say that this organ's susceptibility to emotional upset is possibly greater than that of any other organ, and external signs are often a good barometer of the internal condition of this organ. If we know what to look for, we can easily discover tell-tale signs on the nails, the skin and the hair if something is upsetting the liver. If the liver is no longer able to supply the necessary ingredients for the hair to grow, alopecia may develop and the scalp may turn a darkish colour. The hair may look lifeless with a tendency to split or break. It can also turn grey very rapidly. There is a well-known story that Queen Marie-Antoinette's hair changed from brown to white overnight during the bloodbath of the French Revolution. This is certainly possible and, similarly, when I see a darkening of the nails, I know there is reason for concern. There are always outward signs that show what is going on inside the body. When there is trauma or negative thinking, the liver will be affected, just as we will see a positive change when our ears tune into some pleasant music or song. Living in harmony with ourselves and with nature, and with all the systems in the body, is as important for the liver as it is for other body organs, if not more so.

The biliary vessels begin as minute passages which are scattered through the whole liver, where they select the bile and gall which the liver secretes. The gall bladder itself is a muscular sac holding approximately 2 fl oz. It collects the bile, which is concentrated to approximately six times its density as it comes from the liver. Fresh bile only contains 3 per cent dry matter, while the concentrated bile contains 18 per cent of a much darker colour with the suggestion of green in it and also tastes considerably more bitter than fresh gall. The gall bladder all too often needs our attention and is often very happy with Centaurium or with the Indian root, *Rhizoma curcumae Javanecae* — called Temoe Lawak in Indonesia, from where it hails. In cases of inflammation it can be very helpful to use Echinaforce or an extract of the plant *Silybum marianum*, or the milk thistle. This is a medicinal plant whose history reaches back far into the pre-scientific period of medicine. It is mentioned, for example, by the Abbess Hildegard of Bingen, who lived from 1098–1179 and who summarised the medical knowledge of her time in the form of a dictionary, where she referred to it in connection with symptoms suggesting liver diseases. In the nineteenth century also milk thistle was recommended for a range of problems where disease of the liver was suspected. Milk Thistle Extract is a very strong potency, which also contains some enzymes, which I have found to be a most useful remedy.

Jaundice should never be taken lightly and, as prevention is better than cure, immediate action should be taken if we are dealing with a congested or infected jaundice. People with such problems should know that fasting is helpful and they are advised to take *Lachesis 12x*, together with Golden Grass Tea and Nephrosolid drops. During a fasting period drink plenty of beetroot juice and carrot juice. Also take Molkosan in a diluted form to help the jaundice problem and drink plenty of barley water. In the case of digestive problems take some Centaurium (twice daily, fifteen drops). The correct combination of food is very important and the patients would be well advised to familiarise themselves with some rudimentary knowledge of food combining. An excellent example of this is never to eat fruit and vegetables during the same meal. Reduce your fat intake, and drink buttermilk and herbal teas. Be aware that your coffee and tea intake should also be limited.

It is important to include unsaturated essential fatty acids in the diet, such as linoleic acid and gamma-linolenic acid, which are found in evening primrose or other rich seeds that contain minerals and vitamin F as well. Sesame seeds, for example, are rich in calcium, iron, phosphorus and silicea. In this same context I would recommend Herbamare salt and Trocamare salt: these products are based on sea salt to which is added a number of healthy herbal ingredients and so make a very tasty and useful condiment for food preparation.

Recently I read an interesting article on the medicinal value of berries and I have long been aware of their benefits for liver sufferers. In the article the bilberry was singled out for circumstances when a patient experiences eye problems as a result of a liver disorder. It seems that bilberries regenerate the liver and the pancreas and also influence the digestive tracts. Therefore if bilberries are available, please eat some and remember that no other kind of food contains so many healing forces as berries. From the folklore of the ancient Helvetian and Germanic tribes it becomes very clear that they were aware of the tremendous healing properties of seeds and berries and elsewhere in old literature we find many references to these properties.

During the Second World War liver upsets were commonly

experienced because of either the lack of food or eating the wrong food. My grandmother advised people to eat sauerkraut if at all possible. Although sauerkraut is a fermented food, it still has all the healthy characteristics of raw cabbage, and the lactic fermentation is of great value for the pancreas and for the intestinal flora. It is excellent to eat raw sauerkraut every now and then. My grandmother was quite right to advise this for liver patients.

Over the years I have learned to be very careful with wheat. Nowadays wheat is produced with the help of highly unnatural fertilising methods, which is the reason why its properties have changed so greatly. For some people, especially for many liver patients, wheat has become an enemy and these people should be very wary of wheat, as well as meat, eggs and fish.

The endocrine system also plays a major part in maintaining the harmony of the liver in relation to other internal organs, such as the pancreas, the adrenals and the thyroid. Even the small thymus gland is very important in this context.

Nature is so wonderful and indicates in its characteristics what the remedies should be used for. Look, for example, at the artichoke whose shape is surely reminiscent of the great harmony of nature where everything is in balance, reminding us that the force of nature will always cure.

The liver – the regulator of our health – is affected by any cancerous condition in the body, and is not exclusively involved in cancer of the liver. A liver condition is indicated when cancer of the stomach, breast or lungs has been diagnosed. Although there may be no secondaries in the liver, the organ itself is always involved in some way. A correct dietary approach is therefore vitally important to any person with cancer. Very often the body's absorption ability will be impaired, and problems with digestion and absorption often go hand in hand. Again, the liver plays a part here and we often see with cancer patients that although no cancer of the liver has been detected, and there are no secondaries, the patient still becomes jaundiced. Immediate action should be taken and I always recommend that Boldocynara, Petasan, Milk Thistle Extract or some other liver cleanser is taken because it is remarkable what can be achieved in the early stages of this disease. When a cancer patient starts to become jaundiced we may have the impression that there is no hope left, but nature will help even in such cases if the appropriate action is taken at the right time.

The liver hates alcohol, nicotine, excess animal acids and fats. It is true that oxygen is its main ally. When you go for a walk, try to get away from the city; go into the country in order to avoid the exhaust fumes. It would be marvellous if you could go for a walk along the seashore, to stretch your legs and inhale the oxygen. A brisk walk along the beach or in the mountains is of great help for anyone. This may partly account for the fact that the lowest cancer rate is apparently among postmen and other people whose profession indicates an outdoor life. Fresh air supplies the liver with large quantities of oxygen to help the blood circulation and ward against toxicity. So, instead of taking the car to run a few messages, and so using our legs as extensions of the foot pedals of a car, let's try to walk more, swim and cycle, so giving the body the energy and the fresh air it needs. It pays to invest in our health.

4

Healthy Kidneys

I used to wonder why in the Bible the heart and kidneys are often mentioned together in one sentence, but over the years I have come to understand their role in the emotional body. I have been closely involved with two individuals, both of them with kidney problems. The first was my mother-in-law, who was a very emotional person. Her Irish descendency was often cited as an excuse for her volatile behaviour. It does not matter where we hail from, whether we come from Scotland, Holland or Timbuktu, we are each born with our own characteristics and personality and will develop our own emotions, which make us the person we eventually become. My mother-in-law suffered from a heart condition a good number of years ago. With treatment her condition was overcome and also thanks to a number of things she decided were good for her, because she was a great believer in natural remedies. Unfortunately, as she grew older her kidneys became impaired. Her life was full of emotions and although she tried to be of help to others, very often her emotions got the better of her. She had been a hard-working and strong woman all her life, but eventually she died of kidney failure.

It was quite remarkable how she kept going until a ripe old age, and during her latter years fluid retention was her worst enemy. She kept it under control with a number of remedies and treatments I advised and with strict dietary control. To avoid or minimise fluid retention it is advisable to eat asparagus, celery and celeriac, and with this knowledge she managed for a long time to keep the condition under control without resorting to artificial diuretics. With her doctor's approval she successfully used Nephrosolid and Golden Grass Tea. Nephrosolid is a herbal preparation, the key component of which is *Solidago virgaurea*, or golden rod. Golden Grass Tea, the main component of which is also golden rod, certainly made a great deal of difference to my mother-in-law, and she was fully aware of its benefits. However, as she got older her kidneys slowed down further and eventually this was the cause of her death.

The second individual, the loss of whom I mourned bitterly, was my faithful dog Tamara. From the moment she came to us I realised that she had a very emotional temperament. To be exact, Tamara actually was my daughter's dog, but she was certainly the favourite of the whole family. She was a very intelligent dog, a characteristic that is strangely common in kidney patients. Tamara was clever, and at times she had been known to open and close doors. Emotionally, she was very volatile and difficult to control. On one occasion we discovered that she had killed a fox. She had obviously seen that fox as an enemy, who had dared to infringe her territorial rights. Tamara was a Samoyed and she reached a fairly good age of nearly fourteen, but I discovered a few years before she eventually died that she had kidney problems. The cause of her death again was kidney failure. I cannot describe our pain and soul-searching that eventually resulted in a request to the vet to end her suffering. She had been such a faithful friend and was so sorely missed. The day we reached the decision, I remember that she laboriously and painfully half lifted her paw, as if to thank me for the years of friendship and for taking the right decision. This experience has helped me to gain a better understanding of people who are suffering from a similar condition. Whether human or animal, it should be recognised that as living creatures we experience the same feelings and traumas in life, and the same sensations of discomfort and pain.

This reminds me of a patient with a very serious kidney condition. This lady suffered a renal hypoplasia, which is the underdevelopment of a kidney, usually associated with incomplete development of the main renal artery or its branches. The kidney is small, but complications can occur because of urethral abnormalities, hydronephrosis and infection. Her general health was very fragile and I stressed that it was essential that she took the medication prescribed by her doctor. I supplemented this with some herbal and homoeopathic remedies, but instructed her that salt should be totally banned from her diet, because her condition was further influenced by blood pressure problems. She admitted that she carried a salt cellar with her in her handbag because she could not do without it. When we discussed her condition and the proposed treatment, she had an almost defiant look in her eyes, as if she was already determined to defy any suggestions that would be inconvenient to her. She was a good-looking lady, but somehow I could not get away from the fact that she knew she was inflicting harm upon herself. When I checked her background history I soon realised that my instincts were right.

I remember attending a lecture once and at the time I had struggled to understand exactly what message the lecturer was trying to get across and therefore I had not been able to digest this properly. This professor of medicine told his audience that there is something in man that resists being healthy. I have given much thought to this suggestion and I have come to the conclusion that with some people this definitely is the case, and often there are emotional and psychological reasons for this. Every day I work towards making people healthy and I can instinctively recognise those people who I know will co-operate. Alternatively, I also recognise those who are not going to co-operate and those are the ones with whom I am most likely to fail. One must be fully committed to whatever treatment is prescribed, whether it be orthodox or alternative.

All too often an ailing or sick person will ask 'Why me?' I can only respond by encouraging the patient to take positive action to overcome his or her condition. Unfortunately, too many people sit back and tell themselves that they will just have to learn to live with it, but that is not a solution. A positive mind dictates that you try to overcome the problem, and the stronger a person's mind, the more likely that person is to succeed.

While in my London clinic, I heard a patient mounting the stairs, singing her heart out. I remarked that she appeared to be rather jolly today, and she agreed and explained that she had plenty of reason to be jolly. Twenty-three years ago she had first come to me with a doctor's letter explaining that her life expectancy was approximately one month. She said that despite that grim forecast, she was still around, she had seen her family grow up, and had been able to help her husband in his business. Indeed, she said, she had every reason to be happy, and she thanked me for curing her. I told her that I had done no such thing, because I heal, but God cures. However, I pointed out that she had mostly healed herself because she had followed all the advice she had been given and because she was a positive person she had managed to overcome the cancerous condition that had been diagnosed.

The kidneys and the heart, in their closely related tasks, belong to the physical and the emotional bodies. These laboratories are of great significance in the maintenance of our health, because day in, day out, they eliminate all refuse and waste matter from the body, introduced by an unbalanced diet or a toxic environment. Even if the kidneys fail to work properly for only twenty-four hours, the uneliminated toxic waste can cause uraemia. This mighty filter apparatus, which is put together with over one million mini-filters, takes care of the urine being filtered to the bladder, and its total capacity for one day is 120 pints of liquid. The kidney is only a small bean-shaped organ, but is capable of doing such a grand job. I often remind people how important it is to drink plenty of fluid. Ignore tapwater and drink bottled spring water, vegetable and fruit juices, and herbal teas. Also, the remedies Nephrosolid or Solidago will help the kidneys to continue doing their job without undue interference.

In this too it is helpful to listen to the body because if the flow of urine is in any way obstructed, we must pay careful attention. This is even more essential if the patient has a prostate condition. Again salt, alcohol and nicotine are the kidneys' worst enemies, and insecticides, herbicides, pesticides and artificial colourings can create a build-up of waste material which the kidneys have difficulty filtering. Therefore we need to flush the kidneys as much as possible. Any interruption in the urinary functions can cause an obstruction, infection, stone formation, impairment of renal function or infertility. The urethra, which allows the urine to flow, can become impaired by a build-up of toxic waste, infection or small blockages. If the urethra narrows, the prostate gland is likely to give problems and if this is the case I would not hesitate in prescribing Prostasan or Prostabrit, and a zinc supplement. It is also advisable to chew a handful of pumpkin seeds, fresh or roasted, several times a day.

It sometimes happens that some of the waste material crystallises and this can result in the formation of crystals or kidney stones. It may sound odd, but this is eight times more likely in men than in women, and can certainly be a very uncomfortable affliction. If a small stone were to enter into the urine leader, this could easily cause a blockage. The herbal remedy Rubiaforce is often of great help here, and my grandmother advised taking half a teaspoon of glycerine first thing in the morning, because this often helps to pulverise such stones. I repeat that drinking plenty of fluid is very important as it flushes the kidneys, and also minimises the possibility of infection.

Ample fluid intake also reduces the chance of cystitis. For cystitis sufferers I usually prescribe the herbal remedy Cystoforce. The three main components of this remedy are *Arctostaphylos* (bearberry), *Echinacea* and *Hypericum* and it is recommended for weakness of the bladder or infections of the urinary tract. In very persistent cases I advise that the patient takes the remedy Phyto-Biotic.

With kidney stones special attention should be paid to the diet. Avoid foods that are high in potassium, such as dried foods, molasses, bananas, white bread, boiled potatoes, white sugar and salty products. It is better to eat plenty of fresh fruit and vegetables, while some fish and eggs are allowed. Should an attack of kidney stones occur and the patient is in pain and no doctor can attend at short notice, *Magnesium phos D6* is of great help. Usually, if a patient uses cold-water compresses or a massage, followed by hot compresses, relief will be experienced immediately. If the patient is very thirsty some diluted Molkosan is allowed because this also helps greatly. If there is bleeding, Echinaforce, as well as *Hamamelis* (witch hazel) or *Tormentilla* (tormentil), should be used. Both these herbs have a very beneficial influence and as a natural antibiotic Echinaforce will be effective.

In my lectures I often point out that congestion should be avoided at all cost. Congestion of the kidneys is just as bad as congestion of the lungs, and it often indicates the first stage in the development of kidney disease. The symptoms in the development of congestion of the kidneys usually display themselves as acute inflammation and pain over the kidney region, and some form of treatment should be undertaken immediately, for example fasting, a fruit diet or any of the previously mentioned remedies. Congestion of the kidneys can lead to a much more serious kidney condition, and if this is congenital, great care must be taken.

Some time ago, in Canada after an evening lecture, I was approached by a couple whose daughter suffered from polycystic kidney disease. This is a very serious problem and, fortunately, not very common. It is thought to affect one in ten thousand babies, in whom both kidney and liver are affected, frequently producing renal failure in childhood. It presents a major health problem and even with good medical care it is essential to watch the diet carefully. Under these circumstances the diet should include rice, fruit, vegetables, plenty of still water, herbal teas such as chamomile and Golden Grass Tea and low-potassium fruit drinks. I remember that this couple told me that they had been instructed to let their child drink a lot, but it transpired that they had been persuaded to allow her to drink fizzy mineral water and fizzy soft drinks because that was what she preferred. I told them that they should watch out for this because most fizzy drinks have a higher content of mineral salts and I emphasised that it is much better to drink still water, preferably filtered or bottled water. We discussed the girl's condition and I made certain suggestions. I had a letter from the parents recently to inform me that the girl was doing very well. I was pleased that with some simple dietary adjustments and some natural remedies we had managed to make life so much easier for her.

With nearly every kidney patient I have noticed low potassium and magnesium levels. Sometimes this is because the patient is taking a diuretic, but also if natural remedies are used to maintain a sensible level in the body fluids, some extra potassium and/or magnesium may be necessary. However, these supplements should only be taken with the practitioner's approval.

The other day when I was to give a lecture to a group of practitioners, I arrived late so that I missed the opportunity to listen to the speaker who preceded me. We met afterwards and he told me that he had been greatly involved in research into the benefits and effects of pesticides, herbicides and artificial fertilisers. He was convinced that many twentieth-century diseases are caused by the chemicals and artificial additives with which we surround ourselves. He also declared that in his opinion ME was largely caused by chemical toxicity, and I was most interested to hear that the generally low intake of magnesium was thought to be contributory. I was especially interested because a patient of mine, who is a farmer, had recently told me that some of his cows had died, and that the vet had concluded that because of the tremendous rainfall the grass was lacking in certain minerals, and had especially singled out magnesium. I have heard this theory before and therefore I sometimes decide to supplement these trace elements, but I repeat that this should be done only on medical advice. Ensure that there is sufficient protein in the bowel so that the bowel can bring these nutrients to the blood vessels. I often advise that any vitamins, minerals and trace elements should be enriched with enzymes and therefore using enzyme therapy in combination with nutritional supplements will enhance the treatment. Also, certain kitchen herbs can be useful, such as juniper berries, caraway seeds, lavender, and fennel, as well as bilberries and artichokes.

Aquaflow is a very helpful remedy as it contains vitamin B_6 and magnesium, combined with bearberries – which have long been used for kidney problems, not least by the American Indians. The other day I received a very encouraging letter from a female patient who had experienced kidney problems for many years. I had advised her to use Nephrosolid, Golden Grass Tea and Aquaflow and she wrote to tell me that she had rarely felt better. Encouraging letters such as hers help me to look more carefully at the problems which can sometimes cause irreparable damage. The kidneys, heart and liver are very closely linked to the emotional body. These organs have in common external signs that will indicate if something internally is not quite right. It does not take long to notice bags under the eyes of a patient, dark-ringed eyes or a clammy hand, and I then know in which direction I have to investigate.

I am grateful for the opportunities I had when I worked in China, where I was taught 'to look, to listen and to feel'. Sometimes people ask me how I can diagnose so quickly, but this is not always the case. Of course I do not always look immediately in the right direction and therefore I sometimes feel that I take quite a long time to reach a diagnosis. Yet very often outward signs *do* give us a glimpse of the internal situation. The moment a patient comes into my consulting room I study the way he walks, looks, the hair growth, the eyes, the ears, the mouth and even how the nails grow. I feel the temperature of the skin, and take the pulse. I then usually have a good idea where I should look for a diagnosis. In acupuncture we learn that there are five pulses and if any one of these pulses is out of harmony with the others it is a sure sign that something somewhere in the body is out of sorts. I go on to listen, not necessarily to the words the patient speaks, but to the vibrations I receive from speaking with the patient. Then when I check the patient I look at him as a field of energy and I ask myself where the energy is disrupted or out of harmony. Where the physical, mental and emotional bodies have been thrown out of harmony, health is impaired. The kidneys play a major role in eliminating waste material from the blood. Kidneys not only work closely together with the heart and the liver, but also with the lungs. Therefore examination of the skin will give a clue to what is happening inside the body.

It can be difficult to rebalance these energies and to bring them into harmony again. We very often notice a disharmony affecting our general health. People who are unhappy in their marriage or in their work often have stomach upsets, or they may have problems with the pancreas, the liver, the ovaries or the kidneys. The kidneys especially are very easily affected by insecurity or unfaithfulness in a marriage and such events often have physical repercussions. Sometimes jealousy upsets a harmonious existence with a partner and it is believed that kidney stones are more prevalent in an emotionally highly-strung character.

In the case of advanced kidney disease when most of the functions are failing, an artificial kidney or kidney dialysis has to take over the performance of this failing organ's task. Then all the bodily functions have to be looked at and checked on a regular basis. The other day I saw a new patient in my clinic in the Netherlands. He looked quite ill and his heart and kidneys were in poor shape. He had developed diabetes and he was in great turmoil with himself and especially regarding his religion. Ironically, he was born in the same Dutch town where I was born, a town full of religious contradictions. I remember when I was a child, standing on a bridge in my hometown and being able to count sixteen different churches or religious meeting places, as well as the residences of twelve ministers, priests or religious leaders. This same town produced a very well-known scientist. This man became an outstanding medical professor who produced the first kidney dialysis machine. My family indeed had great reason to be thankful to him because he saved the life of my sister, who was born with cancer. Yet, today, she is still alive, middle-aged and very happy. This man certainly knows about the religious overtones in the town where both of us were born, and he has also been involved in heart research. I know that he totally agrees that the heart, kidneys and liver are three of the most important organs that belong to man's third body – the emotional body. Balance can only be achieved when the three bodies are in harmony. Chemical balance depends very much on the five pillars of health, i.e. nutrition, digestion, elimination, circulation and relaxation.

Another ally of mine, which I often mention in my lectures, is the plant devil's claw, or *Harpagophytum*. The growth pattern of this plant soon explains its name, because it is indeed reminiscent of a devil's claw, and the plant seems to call out that it wants to be allowed to get its claws into the sick organ. *Harpagophytum* just hates viruses, bacteria, and parasites and is also most effective in treating certain types of infection. It is a great cleansing agent for the kidneys and is therefore very useful in the treatment of rheumatism and arthritis. The kidneys play a major role in the filtering and disposal of toxic matter and as nowadays we are faced with so many toxic influences, even in the blood and in the lymph glands, we need to use every possible means in order to help strengthen the immune system and maintain health. I see the effects of such influences so often with ME patients, who have high toxicity in the blood which impairs their circulation so that they suffer from cold extremities. That is when devil's claw will do a marvellous job in rectifying the situation. Remedies based on extracts from this plant are used worldwide. In areas where the people have no access to proper sanitation and whose diet is lacking in salt, remedies derived from this plant help to maintain freedom from arthritis, rheumatism and kidney disease, because the mineral salts in devil's claw are of great importance.

The world's population totals approximately six billion, of whom about one-third live in so-called third world countries. On my travels I have seen extreme poverty and lack of sanitation, but I am always encouraged to see that these people intuitively eat food that is helpful to their immune system – food that cleanses their kidneys. I remember Dr Alfred Vogel telling me about his discovery of *Harpagophytum* many years ago, when the plant was still unknown in Europe. He learned about this plant in South West Africa, where it was pointed out to him that it had great medicinal potential. He has always maintained that on his visits there it helped him to maintain his health. I have often seen him munching some of its leaves, which have rather a bitter taste. He always maintained that this plant helped him to withstand the demanding influences of the heat, without salt intake, because it provided him with the mineral salts required to keep him free from any infections in the kidneys or the blood.

5

Healthy Blood

'That child has the wrong blood,' said my mother when my younger sister was born during the winter of 1944. The food shortage during that winter in war-torn Holland was so bad that this winter is commonly referred to as 'The Hunger Winter'. From the moment she was born the health of this little baby was cause for concern, and it started with a cancerous growth on her back. From there on she was diagnosed as suffering from leukaemia, followed by severe skin problems. It just went on and on. It was the same famous professor, the inventor of the forerunner to the modern kidney dialysis machine, who visited my home to have another look at my young sister. He told my mother that he was sure that her young daughter would pull through, and that from the age of seven onwards there would be a considerable change for the better. This very clever man was right and my mother has often said that the child was the result of the bitter war years, when food was so difficult to get, and the professor bore this out in his belief that the child's state of ill health was the result of an imbalanced food pattern. He was very wise, and probably almost alternatively spoken in those days, when alternative medicine was hardly known. He advised my mother to do what she could to keep cleansing the young child's blood, and my mother took this advice to heart.

The endocrine system, which I will come back to in a later chapter, had much to do with the ill-health of my sister, because not only was she ill physically, but her mental and emotional bodies were also ill. She was a very difficult child with many emotional problems, but when I met her last week while I was mentally engrossed in the preparation of certain sections of this book, it struck me that no one would readily believe how poor a start in life she had. It seemed unbelievable that up to the age of seven she had been critically ill a number of times, and my mother had feared that we would lose her. My mother did everything in her power to give this child the best possible diet, and it certainly paid off. When she grew up she became very active in sport and today she is mother to two strapping sons.

It always reminds me how beautifully the body is put together and how well it responds to good care and attention – as long as we pay heed to the alarm bells. In these three bodies of man we have to be careful to maintain the right balance, not only by being as positive as my mother was with regard to my sister, but by trying to help with the right food and the right lifestyle, to do a good job of cell renewal. I have often been criticised when I state that little alarm bells such as varicose veins and haemorrhoids deserve our full attention. Yet we should immediately check the blood circulation in such cases, for if food is not properly absorbed, and the residual waste is not fully eliminated, minor problems such as constipation are likely to occur. It is astounding how many constipated people I have seen professionally, where I diagnosed impaired circulation. Cleansing of the digestive and elimination system is essential.

My help was called upon some time ago by a doctor on behalf of his teenage daughter. I saw her at her home late one evening and was saddened to see that her arms and legs were as thin as sticks, her weight was pitifully low, she was barely able to speak and only wanted to be left lying in a dimly lit room. Her father told me that he had asked a number of doctors to see her, and yet no one had been able to come up with the correct diagnosis. ME had been suggested, and so had digestive and mental problems. In fact, it was a problem of all three bodies. In the first place I thought that the girl had been mentally overburdened with her studies at university, while at the same time indulging in a very demanding student social life because she had not wanted to miss out on anything. She would take a fair amount of drink, and sometimes she would also take drugs, and lastly a broken romance had affected the third body – the emotional body – and caused considerable depression. She did not follow a regular eating pattern, and when she did eat, it was often the wrong food. She occasionally smoked, because she had been led to believe that it was relaxing. In short, she did not take care of herself. All three bodies had become toxic and were under considerable pressure. When I did an iridology test I could see that her liver and kidneys were affected, and a blood test soon showed a large amount of toxicity that had eroded her immune system, causing her to be in the state in which I found her. What a challenge when I was asked to help this girl, but I am pleased to say that she is now in good health again.

Why do these things happen in life? Is it perhaps that we challenge the body into thinking that we are better than others, or is it, as I have suggested before, that there is something in man that resists being healthy, and something in man not wanting to be healthy? The psychology professed in this statement sometimes plays an unusually major role. This girl, who had given up hope, is now back in good health, and it just shows how the body will flourish if we take care of our health.

Good blood circulation and healthy blood is very important for allowing the liver, the heart and the other organs to function effectively, and for cell renewal. As with cancer patients, in situations like the above case it is like a war: two armies battling it out, the army of the degenerative cells and the army of cell regeneration, or of the cancer cells and the healthy cells. It is a major battle that goes on inside us, and no one knows which side is going to be victorious. However, I have seen victory for those people who put in the effort and follow the practitioner's advice to make sure that the diet replenishes and supplements the body's supply of amino acids, glucose, essential fatty acids, enzymes, vitamins, minerals and oxygen. It is essential that we pay attention to these things and then start on a detoxification programme. Detoxification of the body is terribly important and with this girl, because she was badly constipated and had a major digestive problem, I first of all prescribed the 'Rasayana Course' or 'Spring Cleansing Course', which is always helpful for detoxification of the entire body. After that I used stronger remedies such as CPS, a wonderful detoxifier, followed by Chem-Ex. These were indeed strong remedies, but were absolutely essential for thorough detoxification of the system. Then I prescribed Hyperisan, an extract of *Hypericum perforatum* (St John's wort) *and Aesculus hippocastanum* (horse chestnut), which promotes the circulation and strengthens the veins. I also prescribed the herbal remedy called *Ginkgo biloba*, an excellent energiser, and Imuno-Strength, an all-round supplement. Finally, I recommended that she take some supplementary minerals, namely calcium, magnesium and zinc. These remedies helped the girl to turn the corner and gradually regain her health.

Blood sometimes needs a lot of attention. Life is in the blood and it is often also said that the soul is in the blood. This wonderful river of life is responsible for the functioning of the lymph glands or the white bloodstream. The lymph glands and the white blood cells distribute leucocytes and act as a defensive force. Natural remedies are often effective like the extract of *Hypericum perforatum* (St John's wort), with its attractive yellow flower which beckons us invitingly to use it for our benefit. An elderly lady from the Shetland Islands confirmed this by telling me that the plant itself shows that it is interactive with the blood, because the water with which it is mixed will turn red. It seems to call out that nature has destined it to be used to treat conditions relating to the blood. This wonderful mysterious river of life, of which man still only has little understanding, needs to be taken care of. The Creator of man, who understood the mystery of blood, gave us the laws for it; we should respect and obey them. No more do we understand in the twentieth century how we have to look after our blood. Every time I do a blood test and I find toxic poisons wreaking havoc and causing damage to all three of the bodies that are entrusted to man, I am convinced yet again that we have to make every effort to keep our blood clean.

In a research project I joined on arthritis and rheumatism, I concentrated on cleansing the blood and it was amazing what I came up with. Among my patients I count a few taxi drivers from Glasgow and it seemed plausible that their blood was likely to be poisoned by the lead in petrol. In others the cause may be the tap water that often contains toxins in the form of metals or fluoride, which eventually are deposited in the blood. Amalgam, which is used in dental fillings, is something which I have been wary of for so many years and that too has been shown to be a toxic influence in the blood. These factors must be taken into account before it is too late. Unfortunately, I sometimes see the results of such toxins in cases of multiple sclerosis, muscular dystrophy, or other serious degenerative problems that started as minor disorders.

The lymphatic vessels are longer than those of the red blood corpuscles, and the lymphatic veins are much finer than those of the red bloodstream. These are distributed throughout the body and the red bloodstream and the lymph stream flow in one direction only, with the fluid being returned to the veinous bloodstream after its task is completed. How wonderful to see that the body can be divided schematically into different parts with lines crossing at the navel, and that each of those fields that work on the lymphatic network have a role of their own to play. So often in tests I find toxic material in the lymphatic system, yet this system is responsible for keeping the body fluids, and also the brain fluid, in order.

All kinds of remedies are used to look after this system, and I often prescribe Echinaforce because it is so helpful as a natural antibiotic. If this system is not working efficiently we immediately become vulnerable to bacterial attacks and other invaders which can take over and damage our system. This is one of the reasons why today we see so many degenerative diseases and problems such as ME and other conditions affecting the auto-immune system. Life is a constant renewal of cells and cell tissue, and millions of cells organise themselves together to make a human being. During our lifetime, most of our cells will have been replaced many times in a continual process of repair and replacement. This miracle is accomplished even though cells, and in particular the fatty membranes that contain their living, breathing parts, are vulnerable to damage and destruction. The main culprits are highly reactive molecules known as free radicals, which are produced as a byproduct of something we cannot avoid: the use of oxygen. Luckily, the body has built-in defences against free radicals. Antioxidants are the substances used to disarm free radicals and help protect the cells, fatty acids, vitamins and other nutrients used to rebuild and run our metabolisms. Therefore it is necessary that we regularly cleanse the system, using detoxifiers and sometimes chelating therapy, i.e. Chelate Formula.

Also important in relation to healthy blood is the viscosity of the blood, because if the blood is either too thin or too thick, it will not perform its task efficiently. Think of the oil used to lubricate machinery; if the viscosity is not right, it will not satisfactorily lubricate the machine parts. The most vulnerable are the parts that move, and so it is with the body. Good circulation depends on healthy blood, and on the organs mentioned in previous chapters, that play such a major role in health.

Sometimes minor signs or symptoms go unrecognised, such as the small hairs on the skin standing upright when the body temperature drops. The blood vessels immediately and automatically react, for example when the hands are cold, or in the case of a cold or hot bath. The circulation should be in the best possible condition. My oldest patient is 108 years old and she takes very good care of her circulation. Many years ago I told her that one is as old as one's circulation. I then prescribed Hyperisan for her, and when she reached the age of 100 years, she proudly told me that she was still able to clear the snow from her front door step. She managed to withstand the cold temperatures, because her circulation was excellent. She had been using Hyperisan and Urticalcin, and sometimes some supplementary vitamin C, and despite her very advanced age, her circulation is still very good today. She has had thirteen children, is still mobile and visits some of them who live nearby, can read without glasses, and still has some of her own teeth. For her age her memory and mental faculties are still incredibly alert. In other words she is a remarkable old lady. Every time I take her blood pressure I am astounded to see how good it is. It has always been a bit on the low side, but she has never had any of the problems of poor circulation or anaemia which are commonly experienced by elderly people. Her life has not been easy, but she always kept goats and had a vegetable patch, so that she could supplement her family's diet with essential nutrients, including fresh vegetables. It pays to invest in one's health.

I often remind my elderly patients that they should pay special attention to their circulation if they experience a little dizziness or if their memory is not quite what it should be. Please take note that this is not only the case for the elderly generation, because even for the younger generation a remedy like *Ginkgo biloba* is a most effective nutritional supplement. Ginkgo extract is obtained from the leaves of the tree which, when mature, contain a level of bioflavonoids shown to be up to ten times more effective at scavenging free radicals than other flavonoids. Ginkgo bioflavonoids are thought to have the ability to maintain the circulation of the blood to the brain and to the extremities of the body such as the legs and hands.

Sometimes when I do some soft-tissue manipulation I find that the blood flow is restricted by a minor misplacement in the vertebrae. This can be overcome by a simple adjustment, and we can see a nice red glow coming to the face when the blood flow can take place unhindered. It is essential that we look after our circulation and blood pressure to ensure that everything is done to allow the blood to flow unhindered and without restrictions.

I often see with elderly people that if they have had a little accident or if they have experienced a trauma, that the circulation slows down and then the body emits little alarm signals such as an occasional dizzy spell or they may faint unexpectedly. One of my dearest elderly friends, a very well-balanced lady, lost her much-loved husband. Her emotional system received a great shock and after that she unfortunately broke her arm, which constituted another trauma, which she could well have done without. Her three bodies were severely affected and then she experienced a few fainting spells. I see her quite regularly and on one occasion I told her that it was time we did something about her health. When I examined her I realised that she had become anaemic. She needed blood and blood is a very special liquid. Half of an adult's nine pints of blood consist of red blood cells. The responsibility of these red blood cells is to support oxygen transportation to the lungs, and then to other parts of the body. Every cubic millilitre of blood contains five million red blood cells. The bright red colour is caused by haemoglobin, the iron-containing substance. The haemoglobin is picked up in the lungs and is taken to the other parts of the body. The red blood cells stay in the blood vessels for around four months before being used by the liver or the spleen. We often see in cases of anaemia, when there are headaches, stomach problems, dizziness or fainting spells, that the unnatural pallor of skin will tell us what is going on in the body. Similarly, by looking into the eyes, we may see that there is very little blood present. Good healthy blood contains approximately 15 per cent haemoglobin, which is slightly higher in the case of men than it is in women. The brain is very sensitive to anaemia and in the case of oxygen shortage this often reflects itself in the problems mentioned earlier. Sometimes the anaemia can be attributed to incorrect nutrition, or deficiencies in vitamins, minerals or trace elements, specifically vitamin B_{12}. Often it is therefore necessary to supplement vitamin B_{12} because this vitamin is not easily absorbed and if the diet is at fault, then a supplement is one way to overcome this deficiency very quickly. In the case of more serious complications pernicious anaemia may be diagnosed, in which case B_{12} injections may become essential. Folic acid is also often supplemented and the herbal remedy *Galeopsis* has often been of great help in such cases.

Sickle cell anaemia, which is an inherited form, may also occur in some cases, but fortunately there are so many remedies available nowadays that such problems can be overcome, especially with the help of dietary adaptations. Tissue salts or an alfalfa remedy often come in useful when treating these conditions. The elderly friend I mentioned earlier was feeling very much better when I saw her again recently, and she told me that she had followed my advice to eat fresh lettuce and spinach. People with anaemia should eat four pears soaked in sweet red wine or red grape juice, three times a week. This dish can be taken with yoghurt or custard, and is very beneficial. In the case of really severe anaemia I recommend that the patient occasionally takes a fresh egg, beaten with a little brandy and some red grape juice. This gives a new form of energy, and not only enriches the blood, but also helps to cleanse it.

A few weeks ago a young postman came to see me. In general, it is rare to come across problems with the lymphatic system or the liver in postmen and police officers, who tend to spend a lot of time in the fresh air. However, using Chinese facial diagnosis, I recognised signs that both the liver and lymphatic system were affected. I checked and noticed that the lymph glands under his arms and in his neck were swollen and remarked upon this. Further queries and tests unfortunately indicated that the poor man was allergic to his all-absorbing hobby: he was a pigeon fancier and had about 120 pigeons, many of which he raced. We were fortunate in that this situation could be corrected, but that was not the case with another patient in my clinic in the Netherlands. This man had the same allergy, but his allergy eventually developed into a severe muscular dystrophy problem. This is the reason why I always emphasise that an allergy should never be ignored. There is no need to be neurotic about it, but if there are problems and you feel below par, and the lymph glands are swollen, the blood will become infected and this must be rectified.

The lymphatic system is the sewage system of the body. Every muscle has a controlled blood supply and there is a receptor in the brain for every muscle. Generally speaking, there is always a lymphatic nodule where there is a weak muscle. The release of the blocked lymphatic by application of some light pressure will immediately tell us if the lymphatic tract is in trouble, which was the case with the young postman. Our health depends to a great extent upon this complex lymphatic system, as the lymphatic supply flows in one direction only. Apparently, lymph is propelled mainly by breathing, walking, intestinal activity and muscle action. There is twice as much lymph in the body as there is blood, and there are twice as many lymphatic vessels as there are blood vessels. It is the lymphatics that control the blood circulation and cause fresh blood to irrigate the affected parts or areas.

I desensitised the young postman with the help of a few natural remedies, for example *Harpagophytum*, or devil's claw extract, and also Pollinosan, a remedy I often prescribe for hay fever. Both these remedies are of great help in the treatment of allergies or unusual sensitivities. For the lymph flow I used Lympho-Clear, which is a unique formula containing red clover, liquorice, burdock, golden rod, and some enzyme products.

I am sure that the blood will always remain a mystery. As much as we have come to know about it, I am sure that there is still much to be learned. Sometimes we immediately suspect cancer to be a disease of the blood, but every disharmony in the body affects the blood, and the blood is certainly influenced by what we eat and drink. Looking back in history, we recognise the preoccupation with blood from the scary stories of blood-letting with the aid of leeches. It was on 21 January 1910 when medicine thought that an answer had been found to cancer: it was a virus. On 24 January 1927 Neville Chamberlain, then Minister of Health, said that between 1850 and 1925 cancer had become five times more prevalent. By 1 December 1985 there were higher cancer rates all over the world. I reckon that when I arrived in Scotland in 1970 one in eighteen people would eventually suffer from cancer, while today that ratio has changed to one in four, with Scotland leading the world in the occurrence of bowel cancer.

Do we really take sufficient care of ourselves, bearing in mind the nuclear power stations, which have multiplied by three since 1985? Has science failed despite all the financial support that has gone into cancer research? Very little of the funding has been used to see if nature holds any treasures that may be of help in the battle against cancer. I doubt if we have learned much more about the secrets of the A-lymphocytes, B-lymphocytes and T-lymphocytes, and their significance to health. Have we used the powers of nature to the advantage of health? Although medicine has played a great role in the research of degenerative disease I fear that not much consideration has been given to nature. There is still a great hiatus in our understanding of life as a constant process of cell renewal. We are the living form of the chemicals we retain from what we eat and drink. The connection between us and our food intake could hardly be more intimate. Our food intake is often inadequate or wrong in some way. We do not ingest the correct chemicals to allow our bodies to continue with their life function – that of producing adequate supplies to the multitude of different cells we require in order to remain healthy.

There is another obvious causative factor: the lack of essential minerals. If a certain mineral is necessary for the manufacture of a certain tissue, and the metabolism does not assimilate that mineral, the tissue just will not be made. Again, healthy blood is required in order to perform this task. Therefore nutrients containing vitamins, minerals and trace elements are needed to supply the blood in order to form the right tissue. Blood symbolises life. Even a drop of blood is sufficient to give a clear picture of the entire bodily functions and it is often enough to guide a practitioner to the correct diagnosis and decide on the appropriate treatment.

I think back to when my young sister was born in that most memorable and dreadful Hunger Winter in 1944 with 'the wrong blood', according to my mother. With the help of orthodox medicine combined with alternative medicine, my sister's life was saved and she has grown into a healthy and well-balanced person. We have not forgotten those worrying times and, as young as she was, she still has her memories. This may be the reason that she now cares for people with health problems, because she understands what it is like to live in fear for your health. Good health is too often taken for granted but bearing in mind the laws of our Creator, blood is the elixir of life.

6

A Healthy Mind

Mens Sana in Corpore Sano – A healthy mind in a healthy body.

The mind is a mental state and it is amazing how that part of the body, which is stronger than the physical body, can be influenced so easily, either positively or negatively. A healthy mind will be reflected in a healthy body. The physical body will be obedient to the mind, not the other way round. It is very important that we influence the mind positively, and I often tell patients who are in the depths of despair that the key to their recovery lies within themselves. With a positive outlook or mind the body will get better and more responsive. The mental body is without a doubt stronger than the physical body.

Even during sleep the brain remains active and continues to send impulses to different parts of the body. Although it is no bigger than a grapefruit and about 3 lb in weight, the brain is like a powerful computer with countless parts and millions of connecting wires.

Despite the advance in scientific knowledge our understanding of brain cells is still in its infancy. For centuries scientists thought that our brain contained our mind or our conscience, and it is only relatively recently that they have come to the conclusion that a different approach is called for. It was the French anatomist of German descent Franz Joseph Gall who recognised that the brain had a different function. According to him, the sensors for humour were located on the front of the brain, while the sensors at the back of the brain were for characteristics such as courage, bravery and politeness. The sides of the brain, he maintained, house the sensors for some of the pleasures of life, such as enjoyment of good food and wine. In 1825 Gall published his thoughts on the brain in six large volumes. Gall believed our conscience to be situated at the side of the brain, our vision at the back of the brain and at the lower back the hypothalamus and some of the endocrine glands. He also suggested that this is where some of the mental vibrations originate.

Imagine the fact that the brain contains milliards of cells and that even the smallest cell has its function. The brain controls the impulses to the blood vessels and nerve cells. There has been much controversy about some of the theories that have been published on the mind and the brain, but there is no doubt about the fact that the brain influences the entire body.

Although women appear to have smaller brains than men, this does not mean that women are less intelligent. On the contrary, we see that women are often more clever and therefore intelligence is something that is difficult to define. The basic elements that make up the brain and the nervous system are called brain cells or neurons. Neurons all have the same form and every neuron in the body produces a stream of impulses, even when the body is resting. The outside of a neuron is positively charged and the inside is negatively charged. The receptor cells quickly read the messages, and reflex action is therefore instantaneous – as becomes clear when we get an electric shock or when we touch a hot object, for example. Our total nervous system is constructed from thirty milliard neurons and the brain contains ten milliard neurons, and in the skin there are four million receptor cells allowing us sensations of taste, heat, cold and pain. Receptor cells in the muscles and other parts of the body are sensitive to colour, sound and movement. Receptor cells in the arteries are very sensitive to pressure.

The brain is protected by cerebro-spinal fluid, which also protects the spinal cord. The spinal cord is the most important nerve centre, which sends its information to the brain. After a fall or a knock on the head one should be careful because, despite the presence of the cerebro-spinal fluid which is intended to cushion the brain, it can accidentally come into contact with the skull, sometimes causing cerebral damage.

The bigger part of the brain rests in the base of the skull and in the brain stem are those milliards of neurons which are connected with each other and also with the nerve cells. It was not discovered until 1949 what happens in this part of the brain and that millions of impulses can select important information and send signals to other parts of the brain. In the cerebral cortex there are two very special fields of neurons, which are divided into different areas. That part of the brain, called the sensory part, deals with all the information from the skin. At the back of the brain stem we find the small brain, or the cerebellum, which lies just under the larger part of the brain, or the cerebrum. The most important task of the small brain is to co-ordinate muscle movements. The better known part of the brain, the cerebrum, is divided into left and right hemispheres.

The bigger parts of the brain have two fields, which although divided work in close conjunction with each other. These parts relay hot and cold sensations, control communication in our movements and consciousness of pain. The electrical impulses of the neurons look after vision and consciousness of light, dark, colour and sound. Since the brain was first acknowledged as the seat of the mind science has come to accept that the brain works like a computer, although there is still a great difference of opinion as to how it does this and there is still much to investigate.

When we talk about a healthy mind in a healthy body, we should be fully aware of the responsibility that is put on our shoulders, although a few decades ago brain surgery was already being performed while specialists still lacked the essential knowledge. Even today, our knowledge remains limited and great damage can be done by interference with the conscious or subconscious mind. I remember a case in the Netherlands thirty-eight years ago, when a young girl was hypnotised, and to this day she has never regained consciousness. If we decide to interfere with this part of the anatomy it is extremely important to know exactly what we are doing. Illness of the mind is as old as mankind. In the New Testament of the Bible we can read that a Roman captain asked Jesus to heal his sick servant. It is suspected that this servant may have suffered a stroke and it is only during the last century that medicine has come to realise that such problems stem from the brain. So much damage to our health can originate from the brain, even when triggered by emotional or traumatic experiences.

The most important functions of the brain occur in the grey brain mass – the nerve cells in the outer part of the brain called the cortex, and in the white brain mass, which forms the rest of our brain. Each brain cell is interconnected and highly dependent on each other. Not only can traumatic or emotional interference be influential, but bacteria or infections can cause serious diseases such as meningitis. A brain abscess can be fatal or an infection can result in a serious condition such as encephalitis. Each virus can lead to serious illness, such as rabies, Herpes simplex, Parkinson's, Alzheimer's or multiple sclerosis. Although we realise that our knowledge of the brain is still limited, we also know that we must use the little knowledge we have to positively influence the brain by providing sufficient rest, relaxation and a good diet.

It is possible to negatively influence the mind with food that has a detrimental effect, and this can be done by over-eating as well as through malnutrition. In some research projects that involved close contact with prisoners, I have recognised a detrimental food pattern among schizophrenics, which involved alcohol and a high sugar intake. I have seen previously upstanding people become criminals as a result of self-inflicted brain damage due to poor dietary management. Similarly it is a widely accepted fact that long-term alcohol abuse is a potential cause of brain damage. A healthy diet acts as a stimulant for cell renewal, of which the same cannot be said about alcohol.

During my studies in the Netherlands I lodged with an uncle and aunt in the west of the country. My uncle had a managerial post in a psychiatric hospital and on certain occasions he would ask for help, which gave me a chance to study some of the patients at that hospital. Among them there were some highly intelligent and educated people, as well as people of a lower intelligence. On a number of occasions I witnessed a sudden personality change occur in some of these patients. I still clearly remember that, even at that time, I was surprised by their common interest in food, and the sweeter the food was, the better. Sugary products and chocolate were their favourite foods, and they also had a high consumption of refined grains, especially wheat. Nowadays, as a result of specialised studies, it has been confirmed that there is a connection between nutrition and mental behaviour. In the USA especially there has been considerable research involving prisoners, juvenile delinquents and schoolchildren, which has conclusively proved that irresponsible dietary habits influence behaviour patterns. I have seen many multiple sclerosis patients who have followed a sugar- and gluten-free diet subsequently develop a more positive mental outlook. As a result of seeing such behavioural changes among the patients at the mental hospital, and among some of my own patients, I have volunteered dietary advice for inmates in a number of British prisons. Hyperactivity among young children and teenagers is also often due to an addiction to sugar or carbohydrates, or as the result of an allergy to chemicals, for example certain artificial food colourings.

In my book *Nature's Gift of Food* this subject has been dealt with in greater detail and I have explained benefits of eliminating certain food stuffs from the diet and ensuring the correct combination of foods. The high level of stress prevalent today necessitates a good food pattern, as well as rest and relaxation, in order to counter its effects. The best forms of relaxation are achieved by taking exercise in the fresh air, especially cycling and swimming. The mind and the nervous system will benefit from any form of healthy exercise, which also helps us to sleep better. Sound sleep is also important for the mind and for the nervous system, because when we are tired we become irritable and short-tempered, thus creating a stressful situation for ourselves and for others.

One of my patients suffered from anorexia nervosa during her teens. This is now many years ago, but at the time she was very depressed. She took very little food and the food she took lacked any nutritional value. In a later stage of her illness she developed schizophrenic tendencies, but very slowly I was able to help her by dietary advice and by teaching her to relax and to evaluate her problems. Although this is now many years ago, this lady still writes to me and remembers the 'hell' she went through when she lost touch with reality.

Nature has a plentiful supply of remedies that can help us in such circumstances, one of which has only reached the West during the last few years, namely *Ginkgo biloba*. In Japan this tree is revered as a 'miracle' tree. The extract obtained from the leaves of a mature ginkgo tree is particularly beneficial for helping to maintain the circulation of the blood to the brain. The shape of the ginkgo leaf is not unlike that of the brain, being more or less composed of two sections which are like the positive and negative side of the brain, joined by a little stem, just like the brain stem. The remedy derived from this leaf is also helpful for treating degenerative diseases and helps to improve the power of concentration and communication.

I have seen great successes with the homoeopathic remedy *Cerebrum* in children with some brain dysfunction. A few weeks ago a mother asked me for a repeat prescription of this remedy for her son, because at school his teachers had remarked that they had noticed how his concentration had deteriorated, and this seemed to coincide with the end of a course of *Cerebrum* I had prescribed earlier. There are many different types of mental illness or weakness, and it is not helpful to label people manic depressive, hypochondriac, neurotic or schizophrenic. Only by positive action can one expect to overcome such conditions, and with the help of a professional practitioner or counsellor much can be achieved.

Of course, patients must learn to talk about their problems, and in order to do so we must first of all recognise the condition for what it is. It is no good telling oneself that if we do not think about it, it may go away. The problems may be the result of an addiction or a nutritional inadequacy, or an inability to assimilate certain foods. A very good friend of mine has long been involved with the Samaritans and we have discussed the types of problems commonly encountered. Very often the person calling for help is struggling with a combination of physical and emotional problems, usually with the latter having brought about a condition of physical weakness or vulnerability. If any one of the three bodies of man is out of balance, the disturbance will affect all three bodies, and harmony must be restored. All too often misguided advice is followed and we should ensure that only qualified people are asked for guidance and advice. It was a person with a great deal of understanding who said that 'self knowledge is the beginning of all wisdom'. In the unrecognised book of the Gospel of St Thomas it is written that Jesus said 'The one who knows everything except oneself is missing everything'. Unfortunately, among my patients I see too many examples of people who do not know themselves and who will not recognise that their problem is in the mind. They refuse to accept that physical disorders can evolve from emotional conditions or weaknesses. I can only feel sorry for them because by this refusal to accept the facts, they are delaying a cure. All healing comes from within oneself. The conscious and subconscious are interrelated with our health. God or nature must be given the chance to make us well and if we are determined to forget our miseries, even if only for a while, recovery can sometimes be round the corner. Harmful or vengeful thoughts can be damaging to the mind and therefore detrimental to our health. Always remember that God will work with you but not for you. Man's mind is creative – and this characteristic is to be used for our benefit.

The brain can also be likened to a battery where vital energy and power is stored. This battery is time and again recharged during our sleep, from an unknown source and in an unknown manner. Because we do not know how this happens this does not mean that it does not take place. Always try to relax and to this end you may require the help of an osteopath or a chiropractor, because mental fears or frustrations will affect the spine. If the spine is properly treated and tension is removed in a responsible manner, a more relaxed mental attitude often results, and the flow of messages to the brain is not interrupted. When acupuncture is used for energy balancing it can also be very helpful in releasing a great deal of tension, thus restoring the rhythm of life or harmony to the three bodies.

It is not easy to comprehend the tremendous task undertaken by the brain in relation to our circulation. In the overall picture the arteries rule supreme as part of the sympathetic nervous system. As the circulation flows, supplying the body's needs, with or without us being conscious of it, it is only when the sympathetic nervous system is functioning correctly that the spine can support the natural functions of the body. Relaxation and breathing exercises help to balance the spine and loosen the bones and muscles. There is nothing better than throwing open the windows when waking up in the morning and breathing in the fresh air. Breathe in plenty of oxygen, filling the lungs, and thank God for yet another day. Each morning I think how important it is to meditate on the promises of God and on how to live life happily and healthily. When the day has come to an end, we may look back and ponder on the things we have left undone and how we can be supportive and loving to those near to us. The power of love is probably the greatest power of the universe, especially when we think of the great love of our Creator, who gives to every living soul a promise that Creation will provide food to exist and herbs for healing. Remember, the emotional body is the most important of the three bodies because if that body is out of harmony then all three bodies will be in difficulty.

The mention of the three bodies reminds me of a promising young Belgian girl I once treated. I was very concerned about her and indeed it took a long time before she recovered from her condition. Young people are very vulnerable to certain influences and I have treated a number of teenagers who were victims of self-imposed damage to their health, while they were not even aware of what they had let themselves in for. I listened with great sympathy to the sad story this young Belgian girl, Angelique, had to tell me, quite a few years ago. She qualified this story by writing it all down and her parents verified every single detail.

Angelique had mostly been top of her class at school and at the age of seventeen she was competing on a national level for a top student award. She had many friends, was popular and loved, and interested in people. When she was nineteen she met her boyfriend, with whom she was very happy. When she was about to start her university studies she met a person who professed to be an astrologist. This lady told Angelique a number of things that really shocked her. Unfortunately, too many people firmly believe everything they are told during a session with a fortune-teller, and what started out as a bit of fun can become a nightmare. The girl told her boyfriend that she was very concerned about what she had been told and her boyfriend replied that he did not believe in clairvoyance and that she should not concern herself. As a result of this confrontation their friendship cooled and the relationship was broken off.

Angelique was very upset and returned to the clairvoyant, who said that she had read her cards and could be of no further help. The girl threw herself into her studies, trying to forget her broken relationship and her concern over what she had been told by the clairvoyant. Unfortunately, because of the strain she became very confused and also began to hyperventilate. She again returned to the clairvoyant, only to be told that she was reckoned to have the gift of clairvoyance herself. She became self-absorbed and more and more confused. However, after some time she found that her faith was stronger and she visited the clairvoyant to tell her that she would have no more to do with her and that she was returning to God.

While she was in that mentally unstable state and searching for a definite purpose in life, a friend took her to meet someone with great meditational gifts who, she was assured, would be able to help her to regain her mental balance. From her very first visit to this person she was given exercises to empty her mind. The girl sought to find peace, but instead this 'guru' continually exercised his power and coerced Angelique to empty her mind. The worst possible thing happened: Angelique had put all her faith in this person and he was now able to control her mind. She was totally under his influence and it was as if she were permanently hypnotised or drugged.

When she had been made totally dependent upon this person she was told that in order to join the sect of which he was the leader, she would have to enter into a sexual relationship with him. The guru tried to convince her that she would experience ultimate happiness if she became intimate with him and joined his sect. Fortunately, just in time her common sense prevailed and she tried to disassociate herself. He then promised to make life very unpleasant for her. He touched her and threatened that with this 'Kundalini' exercise he would unbalance her endocrine system so that she would be unfulfilled and unhappy for the rest of her life. Her girlfriend was very sympathetic with her when she was so upset and together they went for a skiing holiday so that she would be able to relax and close this unhappy period of her life. During this holiday, even though she was an excellent skier, she met with an accident and suffered a very serious leg injury. It was unlikely that Angelique would ever ski again.

Angelique struggled on, but the situation changed when she struck up a new relationship with a boy. He was very religious and they felt they had much in common. Angelique thought she might have a chance to be happy again. It was their misfortune that they became involved with another religious sect and upon hearing her sad story, the leader offered to meditate with them, and promised to help her overcome this dark fear that had surrounded her ever since the 'curse' of the man who had tried to penetrate her mind and threatened her with making her life unhappy. Unfortunately, the intentions of the leader of this second sect were no more honourable than his predecessor's, and in utter panic the girl finally confided in her parents who were shocked to learn about the girl's experiences. By that time her mental stress had been converted into physical symptoms and she suffered from severe muscular pains for which there seemed to be no physical cause. Her boyfriend confessed to having similar experiences. They both felt deep despair and their friends who were aware of the circumstances believed that they had been the victims of black magic. Her boyfriend could take no more at that time and committed suicide. In his utter confusion he saw no other way out of his misery and life no longer held any promise for him. Angelique, who had loved the boy dearly, was left alone once again, with a tremendous feeling of guilt because she had not been able to help her boyfriend in his time of need. Feeling at her lowest ebb ever, she started hearing imaginary voices in her head. Her family, through lack of understanding, could no longer spare her any sympathy, and she felt utterly deserted. It was at this time that someone gave her a copy of my book *Stress and Nervous Disorders* and, sensing hope, she asked her parents to take her to see me.

I will never forget the picture of suicidal misery I perceived the first time I met Angelique. The pains that seemed to rack her body would make her scream at times and she was firmly convinced that everybody hated her. These negative feelings were the cause of the voices she heard in her head, and as a result she had been diagnosed by a psychiatrist as being a schizophrenic. His treatment had not been successful. Eventually, a female psychiatric specialist managed to break through the barrier created by the girl and she was very supportive of the treatment programme I had prescribed. The girl alternately suffered from depression, muscular pain and migraines; she attempted suicide several times and felt utterly deserted, loved only by her dog.

I had many discussions with her parents, who admitted that she displayed schizophrenic tendencies. At that stage my main concern was that at every visit Angelique threatened that if I misunderstood her she would commit suicide. I know that it is widely believed that people who openly speak about considering this option rarely do so, and that it is the people who never mention the word suicide who are more likely to resort to that final option. However, her parents also believed that these words were no empty threat, because she wanted to be with her boyfriend and life held no further interest for her. I had long discussions with Angelique and by reasoning with her I tried to help her to overcome her obsessions, and very slowly we seemed to be making some headway. With acupuncture treatment I tried to help her to regain some balance in the physical, mental and emotional bodies, and a number of natural and homoeopathic remedies proved to be of great help: Neuroforce, *Avena sativa*, *Zincum valerianicum*, and above all St John's wort. When I recognised the early signs of a recovery I also prescribed vitamin, mineral and trace elements supplements, and especially zinc and magnesium. The Jayvee tablets became very effective, and from her writings it became obvious that there was a general improvement, because she had promised to write down her thoughts and experiences every day.

Although I had perceived an upturn in her mental condition, the best news I received was during a visit to Australia when I received a letter which clearly said that she was no longer considering suicide, because she had realised that she wanted to live. No longer did I have to read between the lines; the girl had reached this realisation quite clearly and although she was still far from well, she was on the mend. She was still very upset about the loss of her best friend and therefore, on my return from Australia, I gave her the homoeopathic remedy *Ignatia*. Where previously she had existed numbly in a secluded little world of her own making, she now experienced sharp emotions, primarily in her dreams. This was a sure sign that her subconscious was no longer being suppressed into such a dull, trance-like existence, and she was now in a more acceptable stage of grieving.

Part of the healing process involved taking her dog for long walks and, as she also had a great interest in history, my wife and I took her a few times on a visit to sites and buildings of historical interest. We came to like the girl very much. Angelique has now fully recovered and has developed an enthusiasm for golf. She is enjoying life to the full, but knows that she had been very near to losing her mind and her very good brain.

The mind is a wonderful computer, but it is frightening to realise how easily the programming of this equipment can become distorted, unbalancing the harmony of man's three bodies. Any treatment should be regarded from the holistic point of view. In Angelique's case it was her emotional condition that had the upper hand and had such a strong effect on her physically. In other cases it is a physical condition that dictates the mental situation.

Depending on the state of mind and general health, it can be little things that throw us out of balance, and we have to learn to say 'No' occasionally. Follow your instincts to make the right choices. My dear friend, Dr Hans Moolenburgh, once wrote to me on a specific subject and his advice was to say 'No' twice, before saying 'Yes' once. In other words, do not let yourself be pushed into a corner, we have the freedom of choice, but use it carefully. He pointed out in his letter that when we are young, we are like a faithful family dog. We jump at the chance to be taken out for a walk, hopefully to explore new territories, but when we grow older we become more like cats, philosophically staring into space and following our own instincts. Cats are selfish in that they come and go as they please, they take from life and only give when it suits them. Life is lived at a much accelerated pace nowadays and this brings with it new philosophies and standards. Study them and be selective in what suits or does not suit you. Be your own conscience, because only you will know what is right or wrong for you.

Another female patient of mine had struggled for some time before she called on me for help. As a result of a stressful situation in her private life she had become somewhat neurotic: initially she had imagined hearing footsteps in the hall, then she claimed to hear frequent knocking on the door, and finally she became obsessed because she felt that she was constantly being observed by someone standing by her bed when she was trying to sleep. Her mind never allowed her to relax and she became extremely fatigued, emotionally and physically. She felt that she could not even go to the bathroom without the presence of someone or something. She felt haunted in her own house and was extremely harassed. The sad thing was that because all this took place in her mind, there was no way of escaping this threat. I had long discussions with her and gave her some natural remedies, and although it did not happen overnight, she slowly came to realise that her fears were imaginary and eventually became her old self again.

As with our body, we can influence our mind positively or negatively, and once we have allowed a negative thought to become rooted in our mind, it can become engraved there as if it were a reality. We need to understand that the mind can play tricks on us, and with that realisation we will achieve more control. This control can be advantageously influenced by mental exercises, a healthy food pattern, acupuncture treatment, and homoeopathic or natural remedies.

I was pleased to be given a leaflet, published by the Department of Health, entitled 'Drugs alter your body and change your mind'. Don't let anyone tell you that soft drugs are harmless, because most drugs have side-effects. These side-effects can be dangerous and even fatal, especially if you mix drugs or take them regularly. The leaflet goes on to say that if you are depressed, anxious or aggressive, drugs will not solve the problem. Far from it, in all likelihood drugs will exacerbate any existing problems.

In the UK alone more than one hundred thousand deaths per year are claimed to be related to smoking. During 1992 over six hundred people were killed in alcohol-related road accidents. I have no accurate figures for drug-related deaths, but we only need to read the daily newspaper to know that these happen very frequently.

Sometimes at the end of the day, when I go home in the evening, I let my thoughts go over the events of that day and I ponder on some of the misery I have seen. Immorality and degradation has become common because people have lost their sense of life. I often think of the work I once shared with Dr Vogel. One pleasant evening we were walking in the Swiss Alps and looking at the beauty of nature. In such an imposing landscape one feels very small. One starts to wonder about the overall picture of life and the role that mankind plays. In the stillness of these mountains I mentioned to Dr Vogel the biblical expression 'What is man that Thou art mindful of him? For Thou hast made him a little lower than the angels, but hast crowned him with glory and honour.'

7

Healthy Nerves

During lectures I often compare the nervous system with the battery of a car. A car battery has a positive and a negative – a plus and a minus. In the middle of the battery there is a zone where nothing happens: the so-called neutral zone. In America this is called the neuter zone. Positive always looks for negative, and vice versa, which is a comforting thought. I always tell my patients that if they have a negative thought, it should always be replaced with a positive thought. In the end you will find that positive will always win.

The nervous system governs all voluntary movement and all bodily sensations, whilst the sympathetic nervous system keeps a check on all the automatic functions of moving the body. The parasympathetic nervous system is in control of the tubing which makes up our circulatory system, the blood and the lymph. Nerve impulses, according to a specialist at the Harvard School of Medicine, are known as electrical energy. The nerves operate by electrical impulses and the eyes are photo-electric cells, capturing and converting rays of light. The ears are audio-electric cells. The muscles are internal combustion motors, or a type of electrical motor far advanced of anything that man has ever made. The spinous processes are all in the line of the central nervous system or the neutral pole. About one inch on either side of the spinous processes in between the transverse processes lies the sympathetic nervous system – the positive pole. About three inches on either side of the spinous process and between the transfer processes lies the parasympathetic nervous system – the negative pole. Man has been endowed with internal motors and these are energetically whirling throughout the entire body, and are also located in the spinous areas, the negative pole.

The spine and spinal fluid play an influential role in the endocrine glands. The pineal gland, which is situated in the crown of the head, and the pituitary, which lies behind the brow, controls the first cervical vertebra. The thyroid in the throat controls the third cervical vertebra. The thymus links up with the heart and the seventh cervical vertebra. The adrenals, connected with the solar plexus, control the eighth dorsal. The spleen and the pancreas control the first lumbar vertebra, and the gonads control the coccyx.

All life functions are of positive or negative polarity. Any excess is nearly always at the negative pole, and this is when a person needs help to restore the body balance. The osteopathic technique I use is called the perinial technique, which I was taught by my well-known friend and colleague, Dr Leonard Allan. Intelligent use of the perinial technique balances the energy field. It is the impulse behind the circulation that helps to relieve spasticity and congestion in the body. As we all know, fresh blood heals. If we take care of the negative pole of the sympathetic nervous system, it immediately reacts to the positive pole. The positive pole dominates only when it can deliver the current but it always depends on the negative pole. Only when the sympathetic nervous system is operating properly can the spine maintain the natural functions of the body.

The artery always rules supreme in the sympathetic nervous system, as the circulation flows, supplying the body needs, with or without one being conscious of it. Not only can a practitioner help with these techniques, but you can help yourself. You can learn to apply slight pressure with the hands and especially the thumbs, moving them in the right direction. This is the reason that reflexologists and aromatherapists can achieve so much, but patients can also do it for themselves. My book *Body Energy*, contains a number of methods and techniques on how each person can work with these systems.

The other day, after a full day's work, I had to wait at the airport for more than two hours for a flight. I felt very tired, to the point of being depressed. I withdrew to a quiet corner where I placed my left hand on my forehead, my right hand on the back of my head, where the occiput joins the neck, and for a few minutes concentrated on breathing deeply into the stomach and out through the mouth. With such a simple act it is possible to restore balance to the body.

In the nervous system, which is so intricate and complex, even little things can cause changes. If allowed to go unchecked, what were initially small disorders can easily grow into major problems. The nervous system sometimes needs very little help, while at other times it needs much more help. When I worked in Switzerland, I sometimes watched the farmers bringing in the harvest. I noticed that in some instances they would only take the tops of the oats and, when I asked the reason for this, I learned that these were steeped in brandy, and stored for medicinal purposes. If you were especially tired or nervous, and unable to sleep, this cocktail would be brought out of the cupboard and used very effectively. Based on the principle of preserving the properties of the oats, Dr Vogel produced a herbal remedy called *Avena sativa*, which is an oat extract. Alternatively, a bowl of porridge for breakfast provides a great start to the day, much better than fried eggs and bacon. Often, when I have a depressed or highly strung patient, I enquire about the diet, and usually I learn that it has no structure or balance and therefore his or her condition is mostly self-induced.

Nutrition and mental behaviour have much in common, which is often confirmed in patients who struggle to cope with life and are susceptible to nervous breakdown. I am often asked what exactly a nervous breakdown is. I see this as a situation where the three bodies of man are in turmoil. A nervous breakdown can be caused by relatively small influences, or alternatively by great traumas. In the case of depression there is a decrease of body fluids outside the cells and an increase of sodium within the cells, usually resulting in lowered concentration. A little disturbance in this cellular system can cause problems of stress and alter the way the body displays its intelligence. It could also be affected by an inherited factor. If I apply this theory to the girl described in the previous chapter, Angelique, her experiences resulted in depression and major disruption of her endocrine system. Depression, which is essentially a mental influence, can result in very real physical symptoms, such as painful joints, constipation, sexual problems, hallucinations, melancholy, agitation and hypermania, and if this condition goes unrecognised, it can lead to manic depression and even attempted suicide. Prevention is better than cure. When certain nervous tendencies are noticed, they should be dealt with, and to do this effectively always check the diet first, and with the further help of some natural remedies, more serious problems can be avoided.

The nervous system is a remarkable network, in which millions of nerve cells are active in receiving and transmitting information, and it is quite impossible to comprehend how such a system can cope with so much. Microscopic cells, which provide information about temperature, taste, vision and sound, inhabit the central nervous system, from the brain, the spinal fluid, and the peripheral nervous system, to its roots in the brain and the vertebrae. The central nervous system has forty-three pairs of nerves; thirty-one of them are spinal nerves and the remaining twelve are cranial nerves. The sensory nerve cells stimulate the entire body through the central nervous system, whilst the motor nerve cells send the messages to the muscles from the brain, via the spinal fluid.

As the entire body is built from cells, and the nervous system is no exception, human beings are all roughly of the same form and structure. The nerve tissue of the autonomic nervous system is in charge of the informative system. Throughout the entire body, impulses which are conducted via special cells – the neurons – react to external changes, such as a drop or increase in temperature. With amazing speed these impulses move, measured at some 116 metres per second. These signals move to the sensory nerve tissue. Bones and muscles are involved in the wonderful task performed by the nervous system. In osteopathy we are familiar with the nerves of the sympathetic nervous system, where the sympathetic cells lie in the spinal fluid, the chest and the lumbar area, and where the nerves from the parasympathetic system come from the cells in the sacral spinal fluid in the brain stem. Knowledge of the whereabouts of these links allows us to successfully practise cranial osteopathy. The nervous system is so complex that any disharmony or irregularity may result in some kind of stress or nervous disorder. All through the ages the nervous system has been a worry to medicine, and over the centuries there have been many different schools of thought, each with its own different approach.

A few years ago I was invited to the USA for a lecture tour. During the tour the name of a certain doctor was mentioned a number of times, and I was told that he had proved to be of tremendous help for nervous and highly strung people. He even managed to help people suffering nervous breakdowns and who had suicidal tendencies, and in the field of alternative medicine he had a great reputation. When I finally met him in Los Angeles I enquired about his treatment methods, but quite surprisingly he was secretive about his approach. Fortunately, luck was with me, and at a formal dinner one evening, held for the participants and contributors to the symposium, I was seated across the table from him. We struck up a general conversation, but he had not changed his mind and would not divulge any details about his methods. However, as the evening wore on, his tongue loosened as he seemed to like the wine that was served at the dinner, while I refrained from taking any alcohol. After dinner he became more forthcoming and decided that he would let me into his secret, seeing that I had come from as far away as Scotland, and could not possibly be a threat to him. He entrusted me with his secrets and confided that the injections he gave to most of his patients contained an extract of *Radix valerianae*. I allowed myself a chuckle because valerian has certainly been known for many centuries and he made it sound as if it was his own discovery. History tells us that Hippocrates, the Father of Medicine, was visited by Plato, and they discussed the fact that the world was under-populated. Hippocrates' recommendation to Plato was to give valerian to the women, because it would keep them quiet and servile, with the result that they would be content to bear more children.

Stress can be deployed either positively or negatively. A call of distress should never be ignored because many physical problems can develop from a stressful situation, and I have come across this even with serious conditions such as cancer. It is thought that many cases of cancer are triggered by unhappiness, discontentment, resentment, jealousy, a broken marriage and so on. However, stress responds well to relaxation – but however, it must first be recognised before something can be done. Rest, good food and general relaxation is within the reach of most people and this is the most sensible way to overcome stress.

I briefly discussed stress and anxiety during a recent radio programme and the following week I counted hundreds of letters on my desk, written in reaction to this programme. By far the majority of the problems appeared to be symptomised by common complaints such as restlessness, lack of sleep, too much smoking and drinking, watching too much television too late into the night, hyperventilation, stiffness, stomach problems and lack of self-control. It was interesting because from some of the letters it became clear that the writer had realised with hindsight that the initial problem had been stress. This had been allowed to develop into anxiety, phobia, obsession, allergy, anorexia or bulimia, hysterics, depression, fear and many other symptoms.

What can we do when these problems creep into our lives? I had a female patient who provided me with a long list of her symptoms, and she sounded as if there was not much that was actually right with her. It had started initially when she had become slightly overworked, and this had affected her stomach and bowels, which in turn caused constipation. She put up with this, but then she developed insomnia. When the stomach and bowels are not working properly, the circulation is often involved and this takes its toll on the nervous system. I prescribed Jayvee tablets, a combination remedy of several herbs, vitamins and minerals, to help with the tension. To help her sleep I gave her Dormeasan, and I advised her on a sensible diet which would help her overcome her constipation problems. Her physical problems soon responded, which in turn eased her mind and she became more optimistic and lively. Within three months she had reverted to being a more balanced and capable person. Among the simple dietary changes she had made was to reduce her intake of sugar, and she also began to eat porridge for breakfast. Indeed it is true: we are what we eat. We can certainly see and feel the difference when we change our diet.

The other day I received a letter asking for my advice. The lady who had written the letter had listed her health problems in great detail, and there were certainly quite a few. She closed her letter with the words 'Why is this?' I had been able to build up a picture of her and knew that she was suffering from anxiety attacks when she would experience feelings of panic. She also had eyesight problems, was unsteady on her feet, suffered from headaches, depression, mood swings, clumsiness, and was unable to relax. She also explained that her condition was going from bad to worse and that she badly lacked confidence. She had been variously diagnosed as having problems of the nervous system, or that she was suffering from ME. She had been forced to give up her college studies and had not been able to find herself a steady job. All together this was a sad story for a woman who was only twenty-two years old.

When I looked at the symptoms listed in that letter I immediately knew that first of all she needed the homoeopathic remedy *Aurum*. This was not only because it is a homoeopathic anti-depression remedy, but we find that *Aurum* is very helpful in cases of acute depression. One small potency of *Aurum* changed the condition of this young woman quite drastically and her subsequent treatment included natural remedies, such as *Nat mur.*, to be followed by Ginsavita and *Ginkgo biloba*. She was very grateful and said that she could not believe the state she had been in previously. From her many symptoms I knew that all three bodies were involved and I was determined to help her find harmony, even though this was not easy. Her immune system was in a poor condition but when she became aware of the first signs of improvement, she became more positive and this in itself helped her greatly.

It sometimes surprises me to see how easy it is to run into problems and how seemingly unimportant the factors may be that trigger a general deterioration. I remember a middle-aged female patient telling me her life story. She was born during the Second World War and described herself as having had a happy childhood. There was nothing especially unpleasant that she could remember. When she went into secondary education she wanted to bring her school friends home with her, and this is when her problems started because her parents did not want her to mix socially with her school friends. However, despite these restrictions she rather enjoyed her teenage years and she was an avid reader and an enthusiastic member of the local amateur dramatics group. This is where she found her first serious boyfriend, at the age of eighteen. She was happy because they shared many interests. He got her some work in television and she put all her effort into this. She worked hard and, although only on a small income, she was happy. Her family and friends were very proud of her and she eventually got a promising permanent job in broadcasting. She has long since exchanged her boyfriend for another, and another, and so on. Through the company she mixed with she often met friends in pubs and clubs and she was becoming a regular drinker. She never thought that she had a problem with this because she kept things under control.

When she got married a new chapter started in her life and her career continued to develop. However, she and her husband were both very ambitious and whatever career changes took place, it was never fast enough or high enough up the ladder. She wasn't sure whether it was because of professional rivalry, but certainly neither was happy in their relationship. Some lonely and emotional years followed and all this time she drank more and more. Unfortunately, the drinking led to fits, and frequent delirious spells, eventually leading to epilepsy. I studied the young woman while she told me her story, and I knew that she was still in control, but only just. She was asking for help before it was too late. I often come across such cases, when a situation gets out of hand and the problems just snowball. Alcohol will never help to solve a problem or help in reaching a difficult decision. It starts with a few glasses of wine or beer, to be sociable. Too often it is because one does not dare to be different when one is young. It is so important in those formative years that one belongs and then it is easy to be swept along into situations and circumstances one could not have foreseen. The excuse for a nightcap is not being able to sleep, then two nightcaps are needed, and we all know the rest.

I look at three failures I have had in my practice, all very nice men and all addicted to alcohol. One of these men was actually too good for this world, but was unable to cope with the strain of everyday life. It started with a few drinks, a tax bill he was unable to pay, a few more drinks when more bills came in, and then he slowly disappeared over the edge and became totally dependent on alcohol, in order to forget his failure as a businessman. Another man I said goodbye to for the last time in his life was a successful businessman who liked parties better than business. He had become an inveterate party-goer, drinking his life away, promising me every time we met that he would stop drinking. His liver eventually decided that enough was enough, and although his life was full of good intentions, he was too weak to stop. The third person was a young man with a promising career, who started drinking because of problems in his marriage. I visited him in prison some time ago and he said that he was sorry that he had not accepted my help at the time, because he knew that I had been able to help many others.

It has indeed been fortunate that I have been able to help a number of people in overcoming an alcohol problem. In the case of a young woman with a drink problem, I discovered that all that was wrong was a zinc deficiency. When that deficiency was overcome, she was able to control her urge to drink. We also see the same kind of problems with bulimia and anorexia nervosa, which are often caused by a deficiency, and once this has been identified, such a condition can be more easily overcome. With behaviour or attitude problems, people become nervous or depressed and instead of taking a natural remedy which is non-addictive, it is easier to reach for the bottle. In such cases some *Nux vomica D4* is helpful or *Avena sativa*, or Dormeasan, and many times I have found that *Zincum valerianicum D4* has been the answer. Instead of slowly becoming dependent on alcohol, especially in the early stages, the situation can easily be changed with the help of a supplementary zinc preparation, Ginsavita, Evening Primrose or an anti-alcohol tablet. If the battle proves too much, acupuncture treatment can help to break the habit and the desire. We see that with the great number of people I have helped to stop smoking. Most of them told me that they had tried, but failed. They believed that smoking helped them to relax. Nothing is further from the truth. Nicotine may have that effect, but it lasts only briefly, like alcohol. In the long run these habits are addictive and more and more is required for the same effect. Usually one acupuncture treatment, using six needles only, and a tobacco substitute remedy will help to overcome the habit.

Substitute remedies can be of great help, which is often seen with eating disorders. Someone with an addiction to sugar soon discovers that any fix of sugar only places the nervous system under more strain. We all know that sugar releases energy, but this often turns into hyperactivity. When reducing sugar intake, a temporary substitute may be helpful. People who suffer from extreme eating disorders may be helped with the remedy *Centaurium*. As the name indicates, this remedy is derived from the cornflower. The lovely blue flower, normally used for ornamental purposes, is even more valuable for digestive purposes, for treating indigestion and inflammation of the mucous membranes of the stomach. With this marvellous remedy I have been able to help many people overcome their eating disorders, even with serious problems such as anorexia nervosa.

Often the problems go together, like the young businessman who had trouble sleeping and suffered from irregular breathing and a stomach disorder. The problem for this poor young man had started when he was given a job for which he felt he was not qualified, and he temporarily needed some help because he felt he was unable to cope. We meet socially occasionally and he'll smile and ask if I remember the days when he wasn't able to cope. That is now all in the past. He is more than capable, but at the time he only needed a little help.

Many stressful and nervous patients have impaired blood circulation and it is not uncommon for the circulation to be affected during stressful times. In the first chapter of this book I mentioned the building blocks for health, and that nutrition, digestion and elimination should be working efficiently. If the circulation is affected constipation and stomach complaints are the usual result, sometimes followed by hypertension and blood pressure problems. It seems to be a vicious circle.

I remember a female patient in her early forties, who weighed about 18 stone. There was no need for facial diagnosis techniques, because her face was an open book. Even her lips were tinged with blue. Firstly, I decided to take her blood pressure. This was shocking at 220 over 140, with tachycardia. I looked at her – and what does a practitioner do in such a situation? You hold your breath and pray that she will leave your consulting room alive. However, when I asked her what was wrong, she told me about the nervous situation she found herself in and how it was affecting her. I asked her if she was constipated and she confidently said that she was not, because she had a regular bowel movement every third or fourth day. Well, in my book that spells constipation, and of course that was part of the reason why her blood pressure was so dangerously high. I stressed that she would have to lose weight as a matter of urgency and I also prescribed something to reduce her blood pressure. I admit that she followed my advice to the letter, once she had accepted the picture I painted for her. She stuck to the diet, lost a good deal of weight, and then we found that her blood pressure had automatically balanced at a healthy level. Again, she was saved by timely action.

Another female patient told me that she had followed a very high-protein diet, which was supposed to help her lose weight. Unfortunately, it is not always understood that animal proteins can cause hyperactivity. This lady, as the result of her slimming diet, not only suffered from hyper-tension, but it had also caused her a great deal of stress. She was very nervous and highly strung when I first saw her. She had indeed managed to lose weight, but her health was in a very poor state and this was what I had to sort out – the results of nutritional mismanagement. She had become very volatile and hyperactive and therefore I prescribed a remedy called Stay Calm from Montana.

We should never lose our common sense when going on a slimming diet. A low-stress diet is very important and some useful dietary advice can be found in my book *Realistic Weight Control*. I often give specific dietary advice depending on the individual's needs, circumstances and conditions. Because our rushed lives can cause so much stress and tension, it is essential that our nervous system ingests healthy nutrition.

I remember the day when I was visited by a psychiatrist and his wife. This medically qualified person opened the conversation by informing me that he was there under duress. His wife had insisted he came with her, but he had no faith in me or my kind of medicine. I invited him to leave the consulting room so that I could concentrate on his wife, because I did not believe in negative influences. He said that he was very worried about his wife and that he had done everything he could for her, but had been advised that she should see me. After he had left the room I looked at his wife and remarked that she had been through a lot: smoking, drinking, drugs, depression and generally fed up with life. With a note of surprise in her voice she confirmed that this was the case. I noticed that she still had beautiful eyes, good hair and strong, firm hands, and I told her so. We talked for some time and then we went out into the garden for a stroll. I showed her something that she has since admitted she will never forget. That morning on my way to the clinic I noticed something that once again reminded me of the force of nature. The new parking lot around our clinic had been recently finished. This area had first been raked, then spread with hard core, and finally covered with a thick layer of tarmac. Yet, that morning I had noticed that an insignificant crocus had come into bloom in the middle of the parking lot. This tiny little bulb contained so much life force that it had managed to push its way through the rubble and an inch of tarmac to reveal itself in its full glory. Its life force was undaunted. I pointed out to this lady that if this little bulb had enough strength and persistence, how about her? She stood there in amazement, and she too was taken aback by this wonder of nature. We went back inside and I asked her if she would undergo some treatment to help to restore her life force, and if she could again be bothered to take an interest in her health and in her life. I pointed out that she was part of Creation and despite the abuse she had inflicted on her body, she had still retained some very good features, such as her eyes, hair and hands. She was heartened and said that with my help she would try. With some natural remedies, some acupuncture and osteopathic treatment, she has regained her confidence and is now a very successful businesswoman. Her nervous system is no longer controlled by alcohol or drugs, she now follows a good diet, containing sufficient nutrition, and each day she takes Health Insurance

Plus, a multi-vitamin preparation. She never forgets that when she decided to turn the corner, it was the remedy Neuroforce that helped her.

It is so easy to temporarily lose sight of who we are and of what this wonderful life force is capable, this being the fourth principle of Hahnemann, the founder of homoeopathy. This life force that provided a small crocus with such strength, allows us to go through life and exercise that strength for a healthy life.

I remember being called out early one morning by a local general practitioner who was on his way to one of his patients. He knew that this lady had also frequently attended my clinic and here she was lying in bed, absolutely miserable and doped to the eyeballs, completely unaware of what was going on about her. Her doctor asked me what we should do, because we both knew that she had been through a lot. Now it seemed she had thrown in the towel. I had told her many times that I would refuse to talk to her when she was full of drugs, because she behaved like a zombie. That morning I remarked to the doctor that I was surprised that she had not exploded because of the incredibly large number of pills she took every day. One look at her bedside table was enough to frighten anyone. This lady would visit him, visit me and we could only wonder about who else she would visit. She was totally hooked on any kind of medication or remedy, and she would take anything she could lay her hands on. It is very important that we keep in mind the priorities of life.

8

Healthy Endocrines

Some time ago my wife showed me a few photographs. They were not just ordinary holiday snaps, but special photographs made with what is called a Kirlian machine. Kirlian photography is a special way of looking at the physical human body, in a sense as a condensation of energy. Harmony, or lack of harmony, in mind or body produces many observed effects, one of which is a change in the energy field surrounding the body. This field, which seems to be partly electromagnetic in nature, has been observed to change its form and shape during, and sometimes prior to, the onset of medical and psychological conditions. The hands and the feet, being rich in nervous tissue and acupuncture meridian 'terminal points', give an accurate overall picture of this field. When the charged plate of the Kirlian apparatus – with its own regular field – is placed in close proximity to the hands or feet, interference patterns are produced. These are recorded on photographic paper and form the basis for diagnosis.

Apart from investigating the life energy in plants, food and seeds, Kirlian photography is used to assist in the process of familiarisation and diagnosis when the patient is seen for the first time. This science is also useful for observing the effects of a treatment or therapy. It is of particular relevance when the patient presents unclear or ambiguous symptoms or does not respond to treatment over a period of time. Specifically, the method can highlight the following features:

- the level of energy patterns of degeneration
- the balance between the two sides of the body ('yin and yang')
- the nature and extent of any emotional problems
- the level of physical tension
- the extent of psychological withdrawal
- the general stability of personality
- organic imbalance (correlating with reflexology and acupuncture)
- the degree of the patient's resistance to treatment
- the overall condition of the spine and associated weaknesses.

When I looked at the Kirlian photographs my wife showed me of several of my patients, it was fascinating to see how much we can influence certain parts of the body, but especially our immune system, which is of such great importance to our health. She had taken a photograph of a male patient as soon as he had walked into the clinic. Because of the exercise involved prior to the photograph being taken, a clear aura of energy was noticeable. She then took a photograph of the same patient after he had spent half an hour in an artificially lit room. It was remarkable to see the depletion of energy outflow from the patient in the latter photograph. We also studied a photograph of a patient who, by his own admission, was addicted to watching television, and his energy outflow was very poor indeed.

We then looked at some photographs taken of a cancer patient and we were clearly able to see the cancer process. Finally, there were some photographs of a person who was obviously very healthy, and in whom the aura of outflowing energy was very balanced.

This shows that we get out of life what we put into it. If we follow a healthy diet, take plenty of fresh air and rest, it will be noticeable outwardly what is happening inwardly. So often patients have expressed their gratitude for my having cured them. This I immediately contradict and I tell them that I only treat, but God cures. Nevertheless, there is a tremendous power within ourselves that can be directed towards a cure; if we positively determine to help ourselves, then the body will gratefully reward us.

The endocrine system is quite remarkable and provides some very interesting analogies: there are seven endocrine glands, seven colours in the retina of the eye and seven basic steps in a musical octave. First and foremost there must be harmony. In the endocrine system, if one gland is out of harmony, all the other glands will be affected. The pituitary gland and the pineal gland are very much involved when an ME patient has a low hormonal output, of interleucin for example. The thyroid gland is in trouble when it does not secrete enough thyroxine. The adrenals may be sluggish, or the pancreas may be the cause of diabetes. All these glands should be in harmony with each other, because one less-than-effective gland may cause a disturbance in all the other glands. These glands work like a team.

Even an experienced endocrinologist does not have all the answers, nor does an immunologist, no matter how clever he is. Science still has much to research and discover about the endocrine system. I think that the reason for this is that the endocrine system very much belongs to the third body – the emotional body – of man, and therefore is not controlled by man and nature. The cosmic vibrations that emanate from our environment are of great influence on this system, whether it be a positive or negative influence. A negative influence is often seen, for example, as the result of pollution, and the endocrine system often reacts to air pollution or toxins in the air. This theory was confirmed after the Chernobyl disaster, which affected a great many people, some of the long-lasting results of which cannot as yet be fully determined.

There is a lot of talk nowadays about hormonal imbalances. Kirlian photography enables us to see clearly the hormonal imbalances that are caused by the artificial aspects of the life we lead. Spending large parts of the day in front of a computer screen, in artificially lit rooms or offices, and watching television in the evening, are activities that can easily depress the immune system and also often cause hormonal imbalances.

The pineal gland, the 'conductor' of the seven endocrine glands, is actually the aerial to the cosmic energies. It receives the cosmic vibrations that will affect the whole endocrine system. Negative influences, such as those mentioned above, will depress its action. The pituitary gland looks after physical growth, but is also responsible for spiritual growth. Therefore that gland not only needs to function perfectly for the physical body, but it also plays a large part in the emotional body of man. Rest, relaxation and meditation are its allies, because it looks after the system which is even more important than physical growth, as this is only temporary.

The endocrine system includes the thyroid gland. Thyroid imbalances, either under- or over-active, are unfortunately becoming more common nowadays, and sometimes it is necessary to adjust any imbalance, otherwise a patient can be obliged to take drugs such as thyroxine for the rest of his or her life, which will be essential if the thyroid gland fails to produce its hormonal secretions. Nasturtium is a wonderful herb and is nature's gift to help regain balance in the thyroid gland. This herb can be easily added to soups and salads.

The pancreas is yet another part of the endocrine system, and this gland produces the natural insulin, a lack of which causes diabetes. Unfortunately, I have seen a great number of diabetic patients with emotional problems and tensions, and I fear that these have been a causative factor in their medical condition.

Then we have the thymus gland. It is mistakenly believed by many that this gland is no longer effective after the age of forty, while during the earlier years of our physical development this gland is of great importance.

Its importance to the body is contrary to its size, as it is barely larger than a pinhead. The thymus gland looks after our immune system, but in ancient times it used to be called the 'gland of love'. Indeed, it is true that in the emotional body this gland plays a very significant role.

The adrenals are affected by toxicity from waste materials produced by the body, but also by impure thoughts. Through the adrenals these detrimental influences can also harm the other endocrine glands.

The gonads, or the sex glands, are also easily affected by imbalance. I remember speaking at a lecture in the USA, which had been organised for AIDS patients. At a conservative guess I would say that this lecture was attended by more than a thousand people. At the end of my lecture I had allowed time for questions and I asked how many of the audience had recollections of great emotional trauma, or unhappiness. By far the majority of the audience appeared to own up to this. Not only can the physical body be affected by a virus, resulting in a depressed immune system, but all three bodies are involved in such a case. On the other hand it is encouraging to see that when the person is emotionally in control, how much they can do to live happily and longer, despite their health problems.

A well-known singer was of great encouragement to me recently. Not only was this person diagnosed as suffering from cancer, but a later diagnosis indicated that he was suffering from AIDS also. He told me that he had long ago lost his faith, even though, like many people, he had been raised in the religion of his parents. At first he had been very upset when he had learned about his illness, but he had eventually reached a level of acceptance and had also regained his faith. That is when, emotionally and spiritually, he learned to accept his situation and started to work at it positively. Not long ago he told me that physically and mentally he felt able to sing again at a major event.

In the words of the author Alice Bailey: 'The endocrine system is the tangible and esoteric expression of the activity of the vital body and its seven centres. The seven centres of force are to be found in the same region where the seven major glands are located. Each centre of force provides, according to esoteric teaching, the power and the life of the corresponding gland which is in fact its externalisation.' I have found this to be so very true.

Another look at the endocrine system reveals that a small deviation or impairment to just one of the glands can bring the whole system out of harmony. Then we see the mental effects. From ancient writings we learn that the pineal gland was often referred to as 'the spirit of life'. On the other hand the thymus was sometimes called the gland of 'love and purification'. Another name for the pituitary gland was 'the spirit of womb nourishment'. The thyroid was 'the gland of life'. The adrenals were known as 'the single eye', while another name for the gonads was 'the gland of new creation'. The pancreas also went by the name 'the gland of balance'.

The pancreas is a long, narrow, flat, pale-pink coloured gland, situated behind the stomach, and it closely resembles the salivary glands in structure. Digestive juices originate in the interior of this gland and finally empty into the duodenum, opposite the cystic duct coming from the gall bladder. The juice secreted by the pancreas is a clear, colourless fluid which is very alkaline in its reaction and contains a peculiar principle called pancreatin. This exerts a powerful influence in the digestion of starches, oil, fats and other substances which are not digested by the salivary glands, hydrochloric acid or the stomach pepsin, etc.

With all the endocrine glands, when they are starved physically, emotionally or mentally, we see that ossification, hardening, arteriosclerosis or other problems can occur. Very quickly problems can develop that may remain for life.

When talking about the three bodies of man, I like to explain about when I personally experienced a failure of the pancreas. A few years ago I was asked to visit Australia at short notice. Immediately after I finished a lecture in London I boarded the plane for Australia for a flight that takes twenty-two hours. Upon my arrival at the airport in London I had been told that the only seats left were in the smoking area. I have never smoked and I cannot abide the smell of smoke. With hindsight I should have switched to a first-class seat, but I did not think about it at the time. When we arrived in Melbourne I was met at the airport and immediately taken to my first lecture. I made a few mistakes, although I generally do not suffer from jet lag, but I was not only physically tired, but also mentally upset. Just before I had boarded the plane in London I had been handed a letter that had very much upset me. A very busy programme had been scheduled for me and then I went into the bush with a group of journalists, and it is most likely that it was here that I picked up a virus. At one of the subsequent lectures I started to tremble and shake, and I knew that something was badly wrong. I had pneumonia and was running a high temperature and I was told that I had been stricken by an unidentified virus, from which I was clearly not immune, being in Australia. I became very ill yet, to the surprise of everybody, including the doctors, I managed to retain some control of the situation with the help of hot and cold baths.

The night that I was really ill I used the better part of a bottle of Echinaforce, taking 30–40 drops every hour. In all I lost only two days out of my programme and I was able to finish my lecture tour.

Back in Scotland I wasted no time in fulfilling a promise given to an Australian doctor, and I went to see my own general practitioner. Although I had been registered with this doctor for a long time, I had never met him before, but he was utterly amazed that without the help of antibiotics I had managed to control the situation. However, he insisted that I was hospitalised for twenty-four hours to undergo some tests. When the tests had been completed I was told that I was exceptionally healthy, but it was likely that the illness I had contracted in Australia had caused damage to the pancreas and the outcome was that diabetes had been diagnosed. The condition would have to be controlled with oral or injected insulin. The specialist in question was very pleasant and sympathetic, and I asked him for six weeks without medication to see if I was able to bring the situation under control.

I had lived for fourteen years with a diabetic and I knew only too well that if necessary I would have to accept the fact that medication was the only way out. Fortunately, the specialist was co-operative and after long discussions we agreed on a plan of action. I promised that if my methods were not working I would follow his instructions, as common sense dictated. I started with radical dietary changes and I cut out all sugar. Too many diabetics make mistakes in their diet, thinking that certain foods, labelled as being especially prepared for diabetics, are allowed without restriction, but these often make the body yet more dependent. It is better to follow a sensible diet of selected fruits, vegetables, nuts and some wholegrains. I worked out my dietary schedule carefully. I also took fifteen drops of Diabetes-Complex twice daily, which has as its main ingredient the herb periwinkle, or *Vinca minor*. This is an excellent complex remedy for diabetics and I have often seen diabetics who were able to reduce their insulin dependency with its help. Periwinkle is used as a culinary herb by certain peoples throughout the world, where diabetes is unheard of. I also took a *Chromium* preparation; *Chromium* is a remarkable blood-sugar balancing mineral, but sometimes the body has difficulty in breaking down the natural form in which it is supplied, which we find in meat or shellfish, for example. This remedy, which also includes niacin and amino acids, assists insulin in enabling cells to convert glucose for energy release. Two or three capsules daily of this yeast-free chromium preparation also serves as a great cleanser. I took half a teaspoon, twice daily, of Molkosan, which is derived from milk whey. This promotes the production of natural insulin by the pancreas and is helpful for the digestive system. I also followed my mother's example, who used to buy a pound of walnuts every week. She used the kernels of the nuts in her salads, but also boiled the shells in half a pint of water for about twenty minutes. She then disposed of the shells, storing the fluid. Every day she took a small glass of this fluid. When I asked her about it, she explained that it was not the shell that had remedial properties, but the pale-brown thin lining membranes. These membranes she called the 'brains' and if we look closely at the membranes in a walnut shell and think of the human brain, the analogy will become clear. The membranes of the walnut are of great benefit for restoring the balance in the pancreas. After all, I have already mentioned that another name for the pancreas is 'gland of harmony'. This concoction derived from the walnut shells is recommended for diabetics, but in borderline cases, it can also be used for protection against diabetes.

I was fortunate that I was able to control my diabetes successfully, and my specialist was very impressed with the outcome, subsequently inviting me to give a talk to members of the Diabetic Society, to tell them about my experiences. I have often been able to help diabetic patients with dietary advice, and as a result quite a few have been able to reduce their insulin dependency. However, I always insist that this is done in conjunction with their specialist or general practitioner. This time, due to unforeseen circumstances, I had to practise my teachings on myself.

This experience proves that the endocrine system is utterly dependent on balance. The thymus gland lies in the lower part of the neck and extends down into the thorax behind the breast bone. Sometimes when I notice that people are becoming tired, for example during an all-day lecture, I tell them that if they give a quick knock to their thymus gland they will feel a new alertness. An interesting anomaly is that when glandular extracts of the thymus are given to adults the results can be very impressive. Also in unusually small people, who have not fully developed physically, tests have shown that there seems to be an excess of thymus secretion. The thymus gland functions throughout our life and does not, as commonly believed, become redundant at a later stage of life. The pineal and the thymus glands balance each other, because the pineal gland stimulates all positive frequencies in the glands, while the negative frequencies are stimulated by the thymus gland. It is recommended that in a general sub-endocrine imbalance pineal stimulation should be given, but in cases of over-activity thymus stimulation is required. Both the pineal and the thymus gland are especially active in our youth, and we must consider them as youth restorers and remember this when there are signs of premature ageing. Even with asthma problems we often find that a thymus deficiency is involved and as we live in an age when there are great increases in asthma and asthma-related conditions, it is essential that the endocrine system receives our full attention. Therapies such as reflexology and aromatherapy are therefore of considerable clinical value. Also with cases of menstrual and pre-menstrual tension, there is often an over-activity of the ovaries, which again are influenced by the thymus gland. An unbalance of this gland can be greatly helped with acupuncture and acupressure treatment.

Now we will look at the 'conductor' of the endocrine system, which is the pituitary gland. This gland controls the carbohydrate metabolism, sexual development and growth, and it also causes the smooth muscles to contract. The posterior lobe increases the amount of sugar in the blood, causing a rise in blood pressure by stimulating the blood vessels to contract. It also plays a role in obesity, diabetes, and in physical under- and over-development. The pituitary gland lies at the base of the brain, where it is attached by a stalk called the infundibulim and is enclosed in a box known as the 'turkey's saddle'. When I speak about the pituitary gland I often raise its relationship with the pineal gland. The latter, after the eyes, is really the aerial to the cosmos and it receives energy from all its atmospherical influences. These two glands, in our modern society, are very often involved in post-viral fatigue syndrome or ME (myalgic encephalomyelitis). This illness, characterised by extreme tiredness, which is so often diagnosed nowadays, involves the three bodies of man: the physical, mental and emotional bodies. ME is now recognised by the World Health Organisation (WHO) as a problem of the nervous system, but I am sure that it is more a problem of the immune system. The hormonal secretions, especially from the endocrine glands, are severely depleted and this is one of the reasons that many ME patients have experienced not only physical problems, but also mental and emotional ones.

The other day I read the story of a well-known sportsman, which mentioned cold water treatments, about which more can be learned from my book *Water – Healer or Poison?*. This sportsman claimed that cold-water treatments had finally cured him of his long-standing ME condition. Much had been done to help improve his immune system, but the effects of this are always difficult to quantify. Most ME patients also suffer from circulatory problems, and when mentally and emotionally they get to grips with their problems, we will quickly see an improvement. When building up the immune system simultaneously, they will feel the benefits physically. Finally, the cold-water treatments served to further stimulate his circulation. It just shows the importance of the picture drawn in the first chapters, where I emphasised that good circulation and relaxation are two of the essential building blocks of health.

To gain some understanding of the condition known as ME we must concentrate on the endocrine system and because it is such a debilitating condition we should look at all three of the bodies, first individually, and then combined. I have seen patients who had completely given up hope, and yet they have managed to turn the corner and are on the road to recovery. It is, however, a very long process that requires a great deal of patience and discipline. Helping the endocrine system is equally important as rebuilding the immune system for ME patients. A widely recommended remedy here is Imuno-Strength, which is a unique formula of micro-nutrients, vitamins, minerals and herbs. Other useful remedies are *Ginkgo biloba*, Ginsavita (based on *Avena sativa* – or oats) for strengthening the nerves, and CPS. These remedies are all extremely useful for detoxification, rebuilding and strengthening the immune system. The circulatory system benefits from remedies such as Hyperisan and supplementary vitamin E.

However, with ME patients it should be recognised that each and every patient is to be regarded as an individual with unique needs. Therefore I insist that an individual programme is devised, which may be adapted as the condition slowly changes. In every single person there is a force that directs and controls the entire course of life and where the hormonal system, in its centre of the solar plexus, is involved to regulate this. It is important that every single aspect should be looked at in the endocrine system.

When I wrote my books on the menopause and pre-menstrual tension, I often wondered about the meaning of these expressions. I have treated a number of prisoners, including female prisoners who had been convicted of the murder of a loved one, whether it be a husband, parent or child. I have often wondered how far the endocrine system has influenced the hormonal balance, thus possibly causing a woman to temporarily take leave of her senses. I very much doubt if enough is known on this subject and any further studies can only be to the benefit of mankind. I would often leave those institutions with a heavy heart, having met women who have to live with the knowledge that they have killed someone dear to them. Maybe it was their misfortune that a change, albeit temporary, in their hormonal endocrine system, caused them to lose control over their actions. With this in mind it saddens me to see how little effort is made by the medical profession to understand the three bodies of man. I have met quite a number of people in prison who were essentially good and sensitive human beings, yet who suffered from a physical imbalance that caused a Jekyll and Hyde situation, where they would no longer be in control of their actions. It is high time that these hormonal and endocrine systems were more widely investigated, because much suffering could thus be avoided.

Not only could an imbalance in the endocrine system be the trigger for a crime, but much more common is the resulting stress and friction in an otherwise close partnership. Many marriages have ended in separation or divorce as a result of uncharacteristic behaviour, often suspected to be caused by a physical imbalance. For example, the thyroid plays a major role in nervousness, and also in tachycardia. If the level of blood cholesterol is greatly increased it often indicates low thyroid secretion. A supplement based on nasturtium can be used to help the thyroid in such cases, and nasturtium can also be used in its natural form by adding it to soups and sauces. If the thyroid is not fully functional I would also recommend that the blood pressure is checked. Control of the metabolism can increase the heart rate. Control of coagulation is also dependent on harmony within the endocrine system. The female ovaries, for example, are very closely associated to the pituitary gland, the thyroid and the suprarenals. The gonads and the prostate are also influenced by the endocrine system. The functions of the gonads are primarily to look after the production of sperm, the production of an internal secretion which helps the development of secondary sex characteristics, the development and maintenance of the prostate gland, and the sexual organs, the growth and the distribution of hair on the body, the maintenance of muscles in the larynx and the skeleton, and some control of fat distribution.

The endocrine system exists for the purpose of maintaining the correct state of blood protein, tissue collagen, but we should never forget that it is the emotions that activate the adrenals. These in turn act on the nervous system, which affects the sympathetics, and the adrenals link the thyroid and the parasympathetics. The control mechanism for a healthy body consists of the pituitary hypothalamus complex. The pituitary gland supervises and influences the glandular system, while the hypothalamus supervises and influences the automatic system. The brain contains a fluid that balances the head like a spirit level. The suprarenals give cortisone and adrenaline. They use calcium to build red fibre, nerve and bone tissue, and provide tone to every cell and strength to the organs. If there is a weakness and lack of tone, a fast or weak pulse will develop, or a weak heart muscle, uterine inertia and prolapse conditions.

How can we maintain a healthy endocrine system? It is important that we look at all the methods that help to ensure the health of the endocrine system. Firstly, atmospherical influences, which can be measured by Kirlian photography. The eyes, too, are important and in colour therapy they react noticeably to shades of green and blue. A disharmony in colour can cause numerous problems. Colour therapy has a great future in medical science, and I myself am planning to dedicate a future book to the subject of colour and light.

The eyes are indeed the mirror of the soul. Furthermore, in my work in iridology I have learned that the eyes provide us with a finely tuned analysis of the body's biochemistry and of emotional and circumstantial factors which are hard to determine by any other method. Iridology is the science of analysing the delicate structures of the iris of the eye. Under the magnification of a biomicroscope the iris reveals itself as a world of minute details, a complete map that represents a communication system capable of handling an amazing quantity of information. It is like looking at a magnified image of a micro chip. The iris is an extension of the brain, and is prolifically endowed with hundreds of thousands of nerve endings, microscopic blood vessels, and muscle and other tissues. Each iris is connected to every organ and tissue of the body by way of the brain and nervous system. The nerve fibres receive impulses by way of their connection to the optic nerve, optic thalamus and spinal cord. They are formed embryologically from mesoderm and neuroectoderm tissues, and both the sympathetic and parasympathetic nervous systems are present in the iris. Through these nerve reflex responses, nature has provided us with a miniature television screen showing the most remote parts of the body, which normally cannot be seen using conventional diagnostic methods.

Sometimes a diagnosis reached with the science of iridology may be considered spectacular, perhaps even phenomenal, but it provides us with a clear picture of what is happening inside the body. The study of iris diagnosis has opened new horizons and a new and valid method of diagnosis is now available to us. It all depends how well trained the practitioner is in this therapy.

Through the body's natural X-ray – the eye – practitioners can perceive intelligently and accurately how the life force operates, and diagnose accordingly. The majority of people little realise that every abnormality in the physical body, and every perversity in the mental and emotional bodies, is clearly impressed upon the iris. Through its records we stand exposed to each other as though we lived in a glass house, into which, he who looks and knows may see. The seven colours in the solar spectrum and the seven layers of light receptors in the retina show much of the disharmony in the physical body. Light and colour are extremely important. The pineal gland reacts to violet, the pituitary gland to blue, the thyroid to green, the thymus to yellow, the pancreas to orange, the adrenals to orange/red, and the gonads to red. A good practitioner can create harmony so that the endocrine system will benefit by improved balance. There are many remedies that can be used to help bring about this balance.

From ancient Egyptian and Chinese practitioners, and also from present-day Indian practitioners, we learn that the endocrine system can be balanced in the feet, the wrists, the ankles and the hands. The ancient Chinese found that abdominal areas had reflex pains which referred to certain zones in the body, just as the Egyptians in ancient times discovered methods, using the feet, that would help to balance the endocrine glands. Muscle tone is one of the keys to general physical health, and it is entirely up to each individual as to how healthy he wishes to be, once he is acquainted with methods like reflexology and aromatherapy.

The endocrine zones on the foot are clearly marked and the therapist who knows that the secret of this endocrine balance is bringing into play the triune qualities of body energy, has to learn how to use the thumb. The thumb is one of the most important parts of the hand for achieving a good endocrine balance by reaching and stimulating the zones. Just as glandular or endocrine massage can help overcome exhaustion, so can massage of the big toe stimulate the pineal and pituitary glands, and a good therapist knows which parts of the body connect with which organs or glands. It is a simple method to practise at home, stimulating the body energies, and is rather like recharging the human battery. The positive right hand is always applied to the positive right side, i.e. the right hand on front of the right side of the body, and on positive left back of the body. Also the negative left hand is applied to the negative left front of the body, and to the negative back and right side of the body. In order to sedate the energies involves making contact to continue the flow of energies: the positive right hand and negative left front of the body or the negative right back of the body. Never use too much pressure: do not rub or massage the area, just firmly press with the whole hand or with the thumb, as required. This method utilises the electrical energy flow by touch. Energy flow is generated by applying treatment. The contact between people penetrates the skin and circulates in the body, penetrating deeper and deeper until it reaches the bone structure, and then it reverses this process back to the point of contact. This procedure may be different when using reflexology or aromatherapy, where sometimes the thumb may have to be used firmly to release the reflexes of the endocrine glands. Sometimes that can even be slightly painful, but afterwards the patient will feel very much better.

I was intrigued when I heard Dr Osler state: 'When the nerves of the eyes and the feet are properly understood, there will be less need for surgical intervention.' These words acknowledge how little we still know and how important the endocrines are.

There is a connection between the work of osteopaths, chiropractors, physiotherapists, reflexologists and aromatherapists, in that all practise according to a system comparable to zone therapy, as used on the endocrine zones of the feet. A simple explanation of the results obtained is that the human body is only an electro-mechanism. Miraculous results can be produced, even by simple compression massage. In order to activate the reflex leading to a particular gland, we have to relieve the level of tension sufficiently to create a renewed amount of circulation, then eventually we can eliminate the toxins. I see this with patients who have almost cyclical attacks of viruses or parasites, which cause a toxic condition that immediately affects the circulatory system. Under such conditions congestion is common. There will be better health once we have been able to relieve tension by removing the congestion from the nerve extremities, which is often caused by disharmony in the endocrine system.

Just as man has three bodies, he also has three poles of energy: the positive, the negative and the 'neutral'. Our Creator knew very well what he was doing when he created man. On top of our bodies he put the 'governor', our head. Within the cranium there are important governing glands and it is through the use of cranial balance that we can balance these master glands and directly affect the other glands. This cranial bowl, or the head, is the superior positive pole of energy. In cranial osteopathy we see that we can balance the endocrine glands by way of the cranium. The balance between our feet is equally important in affecting the endocrines of the body, because our feet are known to be the negative pole of our energy. We also have another very important area, i.e. our hands, including the fingers. There are areas in our hands that will produce beneficial results on our endocrines. The hands are known as the neutral pole of energy. The combined use of the head or the positive pole, through cranial osteopathy, the feet being the negative pole, through zone therapy, and the hands as the neutral pole, will manifest a positive effect in the endocrine glandular balance. This I believe to be the medicine of the future.

We should all realise the importance of taking care of our feet. Generally this will lead to less sickness and a feeling of well-being. It must be realised that every corn or bunion and their location will ultimately affect some organ or tissue in the body. In my book *Body Energy* I have described in detail how to use the hands, feet and our head to help these three important energies to influence the three bodies. We see so many hormonal imbalances, which makes us wonder if we really understand the hormonal system. Well, as yet this is impossible because we do not fully appreciate the endocrine system. So much is still to be learned, and using some of the methods used by the ancient Egyptians and Chinese practitioners can help us to understand these systems a little better.

I am often surprised to see how the adrenals react to these three forms of therapy. There is a gland at the top of each kidney, consisting of two parts, one enclosing the other. The inner portion is known as the medulla, which secretes adrenaline, while the outer gland is known as the cortex. These adrenal glands are involved in the aggression or fight inherent in man and each adrenal secretion is essential for activating forces within the body. Each successive use of any of nature's forces will sooner or later pulverise them, but with simple pressure on the reflexes of the adrenals in the feet, it is even possible to clear certain allergies. In this age of allergies, it is easily recognised that our lack of understanding of the endocrine system eventually applies to the immune system. This becomes very clear with regard to the adrenals, especially when I see male patients who are desperate for help because their sex glands are no longer active. The adrenals are assisted by the pituitary gland, from which the production of sex hormones is directed. These adrenals may become less functional with advancing age, but if we consider the messages that influence the adrenals, there are ways that we can assist in this hormone production.

I hope the reader appreciates why I place such emphasis on the endocrine system. This is not without reason, because in the thirty-five years I have been in practice it has been my constant aim to learn more about this system, as I find it absolutely fascinating. Negative and positive should be in harmony, like the seven basic steps in a musical octave, producing harmonious sounds. In music lies the essence of life. As the universe was created by God in total harmony, it is man who has brought disharmony, and even one simple tone can destroy that perfection. As music often reinforces a line of thought or strengthens the various sections within the mind, so can the right influence on the endocrine system, in the many ways in which it can be treated, be of positive or negative influence. Sadness, fear and unfulfilled relationships can all result in disharmony. Physically, mentally and emotionally we must seek harmony. Bear this in mind when reading about stomach conditions in the next chapter, and you will realise that most stomach ulcers and stomach upsets are initially caused by emotional problems, resulting in physical complaints.

9

A Healthy Stomach

I have been surprised how many people have consulted me since I had a book published on the subject of stomach and bowel problems. As I have already mentioned stress and negative emotions affect the stomach and often lead to duodenal and peptic ulcers, as well as a variety of other problems. The primary role of the stomach is thought to be related to nutrition and assimilation. Perhaps it sounds unusual but I believe that the stomach is also strongly affected by all the influences that come from outside.

In Chinese medicine the stomach is seen as the element of fire, realising that in human beings this active part in the body, 'yang' (positive), is acceptable to the 'yin' (negative) element of water. This is sometimes conflicting, if positive and negative are not balanced and if there is disharmony. It is often said that the way to a man's heart is through the stomach and if there is no harmony, there will be acidity in the stomach. Such acidity can be very uncomfortable and can be caused by eating the wrong foods, by eating before exercising or just before going to bed, or by over-eating – to name but a few possible causes. However, very often an emotional condition is also involved in this process. If we are upset or excited, the usual digestive process will be affected by a change in the digestive juices in the stomach. If the stomach becomes irritated or agitated, it will affect the duodenum and if there is a lack of amino acids, glucose and essential fatty acids, an absorption problem will result.

Impaired absorption can cause constipation, malnutrition or poor circulation, all of which are influenced by the stomach. The stomach is yet another technical miracle. The stomach tissue is very elastic where we have veins, lymph and nerves, etc. The stomach lining is by no means smooth, because there are a number of big folds and creases, while the larger of these creases are themselves divided into smaller creases. Enlarged, it presents a picture that could be likened to the ridges in a modern central heating radiator. Approximately five million small glands in the stomach protect the ridged lining from the mucous membrane.

These glands secrete pepsin and fermentation in carefully measured doses, by way of minute sprays, according to the quantities and kinds of foods ingested. The pepsin is only capable of functioning correctly if sufficient hydrochloric acid is secreted. The presence of some acid is essential because without this the pepsin would be ineffective. A healthy stomach depends therefore on a well-balanced diet – a diet that should have the correct acid/alkaline balance. Sometimes there is too much or too little acid, and this may be easily corrected.

During my years as a student I was often intrigued by the fact that in these little folds of the stomach wall could hide the source of potential infections or a stockpile of undigestable matter. This characteristic makes us more vulnerable to stomach problems that can lead to either gastric, peptic or duodenal ulcers. I clearly remember, in the 1950s, when a product was developed that was based on liquorice. This was of great benefit to people who, especially after the stress of the war years, had developed stomach disorders. It was one of the first products that made a real impression and it helped numerous people. The chemist who developed this product explained that by filling the little holes in the stomach lining and closing them off, healing could take place. Although this theory was not universally accepted, this remedy was certainly of help to many people in those days. I find it fascinating that such a simple product as liquorice can provide such great relief for stomach problems. By taking care of stomach conditions, bowel problems will also be alleviated. It appears that in countries where pure liquorice is eaten, stomach complaints are much less frequent. I noticed this when I worked in China. The Chinese have a taste for liquorice, ginger and certain other herbs. Dr Alfred Vogel and I discussed this, because he also was concerned about the increase in stomach disorders. At that time we compiled a programme for the treatment of stomach conditions. Three times daily the herbal remedy Petasan may be taken – five drops before meals; Gastronol, three times daily – four tablets before meals; and *Centaurium*, three times daily – ten drops before meals. We have used this programme successfully over the years and it was found to be very beneficial. Later I added to this programme a remedy called DGL, which is a liquorice concentrate. Of course there are other things you can do to help yourself. In particular, it would be wise to avoid alcohol, coffee, chocolate and wheat products, and to reduce the intake of cabbage and onions. It is also better to eat toast in preference to normal bread.

Many digestive problems originate from an over-acid system, such as stomach ulcers, eczema or psoriasis. Therefore it is necessary to avoid foods with a high level of acidity, such as pork in any shape or form, and citrus fruits, as well as the other offenders I have already mentioned above. Another big offender is, of course, nicotine, and I have come across this as a causative factor far too often. An old-fashioned method for filtering the acid system, which is very cheap and effective, is to wash an unpeeled raw potato, grate it, and press out the juice (there will not be much juice). This should be done first thing in the morning and the juice taken immediately. It may not taste very nice, and is likely to shake you wide awake, but it provides great relief for stomach problems. Very often when people lack the money to buy the remedies mentioned earlier, I tell them that they can help themselves with liquorice and the juice of a raw potato, and they will see for themselves the tremendous health benefits.

I remember my partner, Dr Alfred Vogel, emphasising at almost every lecture, in response to questions regarding the stomach and bowel, that tension and worry should be avoided wherever possible because these are often the start of such problems. If you are not happy at work or with your partner, do something about it, but do not let it ruin your health. Our emotions, worries and sadness all influence the workings of the stomach. I often hear patients telling me that they have felt butterflies in their stomach, or when they wake up in the morning they have a funny sensation in the stomach. All the important organs of the body are situated around the stomach. When I worked in India I was amazed when a practitioner showed me how he worked on the system which he called the organ reflex abdominal treatment. He showed me where he treated the heart, the spleen, the stomach, the gall bladder, the kidneys and the liver. In these areas all the reflexes from the abdominal area are present and we often refer to the stomach as the vegetative nervous system's protection.

I have advised many patients on the Hara breathing method. This involves simple exercises that relax the abdominal area, where tension can be so detrimental to our health. One of the very simple Hara exercises is one that I frequently practise myself. About four o'clock in the afternoon, the time of day when I was born, I sometimes begin to feel a little tired. This, by the way, is an experience which many people feel when the time of their birth approaches. I lie on the floor when I feel tired and tell myself to relax completely. My eyes are closed and I tell every part of my body, from top to toe, to relax until I feel as if I am sinking deeper and deeper into the floor. Then I place my left hand about half an inch beneath my navel and place my other hand over the top of it. At that point, a magnetic ring on the vital centre of man — 'Hara' — will have been formed. The Chinese have an old saying that the navel is the gate to all happiness and certainly, by doing this, one feels very relaxed. Next, I breathe in slowly through the nose, filling my stomach with air and keeping the rib cage still. This sounds easier than it is, and actually takes a little time to master properly.

Concentrate the mind on the stomach and breathe in slowly. Once the stomach is filled with air, purse your lips and slowly breathe out, pulling the stomach flat. This can be done as often as necessary. Normally, the sensation after finishing this exercise is either one of complete relaxation and the desire for a nice sleep, or of refreshment and the desire to return to work. I must stress that it should be performed naturally, as a baby would do it. Sometimes it helps to imagine yourself walking in a beautiful garden where you discover the wonderful scent of roses which you slowly inhale. Personally, I find that this exercise increases my energy flow dramatically and I am surprised how simple and yet how therapeutic it is.

Hunger and appetite are messages emitted by the stomach, and ulcers are easily caused by unhappiness, because some people may lose their appetite when they feel unhappy or unfulfilled, whereas others will start to over-eat as compensation. So often when we are caught in a trap like this, our food is not even chewed properly; yet by chewing food properly and mixing it with saliva, the task of the digestive system is greatly facilitated. Obesity is often caused by ingesting food that does not get the chance of being properly digested. Then other problems will result, sometimes even requiring surgical attention. Make sure that indigestion does not develop into chronic indigestion.

I am not surprised, having worked for twenty-five years in Scotland, that Scotland has the highest rate of stomach cancer in the world. I have seen the unbalanced diet and the little time people take to eat their food, as well as the monotony and lack of variety in the food. The other day a female patient came to me with clear indications of dyspepsia, which is a form of nervous indigestion, that can have some very unpleasant symptoms. I listened to her story, her worries about her family and her family's business. In response to my questions I learned about her poor eating habits and I was not surprised that she was suffering from an uncomfortable stomach disorder. Fortunately, with some acupuncture treatment and some natural remedies I managed to relieve the situation and she promised that she would take more care with her diet.

Another patient of mine, the owner of a large business who had fallen on bad times, developed chronic gastritis, a condition where the stomach lining is constantly irritated or inflamed. Every time he opened his mail and found yet another unpaid bill or a letter reminding him of his threatening financial state of affairs, he would suffer another attack. These worries affected his body chemistry. The stomach and bowels play an important combined role and all that is imported should be exported within twenty-four hours. The system should work like a well-run factory.

It used to be that many more men had stomach ulcers than women. Nowadays (could it be because of equal opportunities?) I see more and more female patients with stomach conditions.

The stomach also comes under attack from a great many toxic influences, not only tension, which can cause toxicity, but also food tainted by herbicides, pesticides and artificial fertilisers. I had such a patient in the Netherlands and immediately I prescribed Belladonna, Gastronol, and some *Rhus tox*. The latter remedy is derived from a poisonous plant, but thanks to this low potency preparation we managed to overcome the toxic situation.

We are all familiar with the expression that the stomach feels tied into a knot. Worries, emotions and feelings of depression can easily cause such a sensation. Relaxation and good circulation are very important for countering this. The other day a patient showed me a herbal extract she had obtained from another practitioner, a very competent herbalist. When I checked the composition of this combination remedy I was happy, because my colleague had understood the close relationship between relaxation and circulation and most of the remedy's ingredients were aimed at improvement in these areas. One of the ingredients was a favourite of mine: *Aesculus hippocastanum*, or the horse chestnut. This is an outstanding remedy for circulation problems.

Elderly people often try to relax the stomach with peppermint. Some peppermint leaves may be added to a salad, or they may be chewed on their own. Nowadays there are some wonderful peppermint remedies available in tablet or powder form, from Obbekjaers, named after its Danish manufacturer. Mr Obbekjaer researched his formula over a long period and invited and received the co-operation of many of his friends and neighbours, and his products have eventually been marketed for the benefit of many people. These are excellent remedies that help to relieve tension and promote the effectiveness of the digestion and the circulation, in order to avoid stomach problems that can so easily develop. Let us not forget that this part of our chemistry should be looked after.

Finally, proper digestion and elimination are necessary, so please ensure that you avoid constipation by taking care to follow a healthy diet and drinking plenty of juices such as cabbage juice and carrot juice. Bilberry and cranberry juices will also help to provide the right gastric juices which are necessary for a healthy digestion and elimination.

10

A Healthy Spleen

I recently treated a patient who had had the unfortunate experience of being afflicted by some very uncomfortable stomach problems. For pain relief he had taken more than his share of aspirin tablets and other painkillers, without stopping to think how much damage these tablets would cause to his stomach. Tests showed that the spleen had become toxic after he had overdosed himself. He never took any steps for detoxification, and before the outcome of the tests was known, he had already taken a good many antibiotics in order to cover up the effects of the real problem. Anything that is wrong in the body must be fully investigated: any symptom that is subdued, or pain that is ignored, may be an alarm signal, which if persistently ignored, may lead to more serious problems. However, I found him to be a very co-operative patient and did everything possible to help him. Like most people, he had limited medical knowledge, and I took great pains to explain the important role of the spleen.

The chief function of the spleen is that of detoxification. The spleen is always involved in toxic conditions and in the renewal of cells. Hyperfunction can cause extreme anaemia. The spleen is usually affected in cases of typhoid, malaria and severe anaemia. The lymph and the suprarenals are always associated with the spleen. Prolapses, ptosis and atony point to low function of the post pituitary and suprarenals, as the post-pituitary stimulates the muscles and the suprarenals build up strength. The suprarenal medulla stimulates the sympathetic nerves and inhibits the parasympathetics. The suprarenal cortex regulates the carbohydrate metabolism, sodium secretion, renal function, maintains body strength and manufactures certain vitamins. It is understood that Addison's disease is usually the result of hyperfunction of the suprarenal cortex. The suprarenals react to blood pressure fluctuations. Usually the spleen is high in sulphur, and its two main functions are detoxification and maintaining the composition of blood circulation at certain levels. If this gland is not well balanced, the brain will not function well either. A patient has a better fighting chance if the spleen is in a fair condition.

This normally cheerful patient was depressed and emotionally vulnerable because of his condition, and he was so down-hearted that the resulting negative influences were not helping him. I asked him if he had spent much time abroad, as it is known that the spleen is susceptible to a low-grade typhoid, sometimes with a low fever or malaria. I also enquired about his diet, because anaemia is often a problem and people with an anaemic condition should take extra sulphur and iron. Firstly, I advised my patient to take Molkosan and to use garlic as a condiment in his cooking. I also advised him to supplement his diet with garlic capsules. Coincidentally, I had just learned that sheep's milk and sheep's yoghurt were also wonderful remedies for his condition. Because the spleen and the liver are closely related, in many cases the stomach gets involved, leading to hyper-acidity, acidosis and general toxaemia, and when the spleen becomes inactive the lymph nodes may carry on this function.

I must admit that my patient followed all my advice, and also took Echinaforce and Milk Thistle Extract. I expected there to be a slightly chronic condition as his spleen was already showing signs of hardening. In an acute spleen condition this organ is soft and flabby. There was tenderness on pressure and a slight increase in his blood pressure. As the spleen also influences the fluid levels in the body and the circulation, it will be evident how much the circulatory system is involved. This patient obeyed every instruction and did everything possible to help himself because, as he said himself, he was feeling very much under the weather. This gentleman, who led a very busy life as a top business executive, had to make amends in his lifestyle.

I could not help comparing him to another patient of mine, who also worked under great pressure, in an artificially lit room, and had been subjected to slight radiation. His spleen had become diseased as a result. The persistent fear and worry had thrown the endocrine system completely out of balance and tests showed that he had become a diabetic. We managed to determine that the diabetes was caused by the posterior pituitary gland, and that his pineal gland was involved. This was probably because the pineal gland – the aerial of the body – had been over-exposed to artificial light. He then suffered the embarrassing problem of bedwetting – enuresis – and low functioning of the suprarenals. Then he became asthmatic, and developed further respiratory problems. Although I did everything I could to help him, he was not able to pull through. His immune system had suffered so badly that there was nothing anyone could do. I had grown very fond of him and together with his doctor and specialist we did all we could, but it was too late. We must never forget that when the spleen becomes involved, immediate action is always necessary.

Problems with the spleen can cause complications during pregnancy, because the placental secretion cannot hold the menstrual secretion in check. The placenta then helps itself and in some cases there is a spontaneous miscarriage. The hyperfunction of the posterior pituitary also plays a very important part here. Sometimes the functions of the posterior pituitary gland stay too high and those of the thyroid too low, and the result is a tendency to high blood pressure, so it is necessary to keep a very close eye on the pancreas. During the menopause it may be advisable to have the sympathetic nervous system checked at regular intervals. As the spleen is the governing gland of the lymphatic system, it has an important role to play in the detoxification of all the waste material that enters into the system. When immunity in the body is depleted, and the system becomes more toxic, a highly toxic condition may develop, when antibiotics must be administered. In anaemic conditions all kinds of problems can arise, for example, enlargement of the spleen or fever, and the patient often complains that they cannot cope. With any spleen condition medical advice should be sought and a doctor or specialist who is willing to co-operate with a qualified naturopath would be the best choice. A naturopathic practitioner will be very helpful because fasting, dieting and detoxification is always beneficial, and introducing a good dietary regime may even be instrumental in avoiding the removal of the spleen.

It is also important to strengthen the immune system as the structure and function of the spleen can be divided into two parts: the part playing a role in the immune system is represented by the white pulp, and the venous sinuses are represented by the red pulp. The white pulp generates the protective antibodies, influencing the immune system, E-, A-, and T-lymphocytes and plasma cells in the lymphoid organs. The red pulp looks after the removal of unwanted matter and bacteria. With ME patients I have often seen that the spleen is involved if the blood circulation has become sluggish and is carrying too much waste and toxic material. A cleansing diet, including plenty of fruit and vegetable juices, will be helpful here, or the diet I have recommended for the liver. For a low blood count Vitaforce together with Urticalcin should be taken, along with Petasan, which is derived from the the butterbur and acts as a cell renewer. In cases where the spleen is enlarged use a combination of

Echinaforce, *Arnica D4* and Nephrosolid. Galeopsis is also recommended for this purpose. Once again I must stress that, as the spleen plays an essential role in the body, one must take professional advice.

I have already mentioned the possibility of anaemia and where this occurs minerals such as iron and zinc should be supplemented. Every mineral in our body comes from the food that we have eaten. Minerals, many of which are metals, all originate in the soil and are taken up by plants which are then eaten by us. Vitamins, on the other hand, do not come from the soil but are synthesised by plants. Although minerals cannot be destroyed by cooking, as can vitamins, they can easily be lost from our food: in the case of vegetables, by peeling or by boiling in water, and in the case of rice and cereals, by polishing. Modern diets, which are high in starchy and fatty foods, are known to be low in minerals. Minerals can be split into two main groups, macrominerals and trace elements, according to the amount required by our bodies. For example, a 70 kg man has 1.7 kg of calcium in his body, but only 50 mg of iodine. Both are essential, but one is present at levels 34,000 times higher than the level of the other.

The most common minerals are listed below:

Macrominerals	*Trace elements*
Calcium	Zinc
Magnesium	Selenium
Sodium	Iodine
Chlorine	Iron
Phosphorus	Manganese
Potassium	Chromium

Iron is one of the nutrients most commonly lacking among women, since the iron contained in red blood cells is lost during menstruation. Iron plays a vital role since it is necessary for the transportation of oxygen around our bodies. It is also a component of the proteins needed for the blood and muscles. It is most readily obtained from meat, particularly liver, so vegetarians and anyone who eats little red meat should take extra care to ensure that their iron intake is adequate.

Zinc is a trace element that is involved in hundreds of metabolic reactions and is also co-factor to more than eighty enzymes in the body. Up to 20 per cent of the zinc in our bodies is found in the skin, where it is instrumental in maintaining a healthy complexion. Zinc is also required for:

- healthy growth through its role in the synthesis of DNA and protein
- its role in maintaining the immune system
- maintaining the balance of blood sugar through insulin
- maintaining a healthy liver
- maintaining our sense of smell, taste and vision
- the healthy functioning of the reproductive organs, particularly in men since it is a component of semen.

Many nutritionists believe that people find it more difficult to obtain sufficient zinc in their diet than any other mineral because its natural levels are depleted by modern agriculture and food processing methods. Foods rich in zinc include red meat, eggs and fish. Vegetables contain lower amounts of zinc and sometimes this is bound up with indigestable fibre, thus further reducing the value of vegetables as a source of zinc. This is why vegetarians and vegans often choose to supplement with zinc, as do smokers, drinkers, the elderly and athletes – the latter because zinc is lost in perspiration.

Depending on the severity of the condition I might also prescribe Imuno-Strength. I repeat that detoxification is very important and in this connection I would like to mention a remedy I learned about within the last two years, a remedy called CPS. I believe that this is probably one of the best detoxification remedies I have ever come across. It is a combination remedy designed as a Cellular Protection System, hence the name CPS, and it contains the highest concentration of antioxidant nutrients in a base of unique herbal extracts and other natural compounds. Beta carotene, vitamin E, vitamin C, selenium, zinc and manganese all have antioxidant functions. Riboflavin helps regenerate antioxidants after they have neutralised free radicals. This super-antioxidant complex also provides pycnogenols derived from grape seeds and green tea extract. These substances are 50–200 times more potent than vitamin E. Curcumin, the yellow pigment obtained from the Asian plant curcuma, and N-acetylcysteine, a stable form of the essential amino acid cysteine, are also powerful antioxidants. CPS also supplies concentrated extracts of cabbage, garlic, ginger and Klamath blue-green algae, all of which contain a broad range of antioxidant nutrients. In summary, CPS is the most comprehensive antioxidant formula available and some of my patients have greatly benefited from this remedy.

When the spleen is affected and there is a fever, the patient is usually prescribed antibiotics. It is sometimes helpful for a natural antibiotic to be taken prior to surgery. I remember a patient in the Netherlands whose religion forbade the use of any kind of medication, even homoeopathic remedies. With great effort I managed to persuade him to take the medicine that his specialist had prescribed, because it was desperately necessary. I then mentioned the need to take a natural antibiotic, and found that he did not believe that such a remedy was available. I suggested that he probably knew his Bible better than I did, but from my scientific background I knew that more than three thousand years ago King David was aware of the benefits of a natural antibiotic, when he wrote Psalm 51: 'Wash me with hyssop, and I shall be whiter than snow.' He knew that his body was being punished for the dreadful sins he had committed, and he needed healing. He also knew when he mentioned that he wanted to be washed with hyssop, that on the top of this plant a fungal growth often appears, which acts as a natural antibiotic. I told my patient that he could take hyssop together with Echinaforce, which is a stronger antibiotic. However, my patient struggled with his conscience and found it impossible to accept his illness. We often find that in a crisis people refuse to accept their problem, because emotionally and spiritually they fail to grasp reality. Overpowering enemies such as bacteria, viruses, toxins and parasites cause a major battle within the body, and in the next chapter I will explain that the bowels of man are often involved in such a great battle, which invariably affects other important parts of the body.

11

Healthy Bowels

It is now more than thirty-five years since Dr Vogel and I opened the first clinic for natural medicine in the Netherlands. I have come to know and appreciate Dr Vogel as a man of great knowledge, and I am grateful for the opportunities I have had in life. He counts as one the two most influential tutors I have had, the other being Dr Leonard Allan, and I have the highest regard for both men. They have shown great vision and as they both worked independently towards that vision, during their lifetime they have witnessed great changes. At the time of writing this book, they are both still alive, albeit at a ripe old age. Whenever we meet it is impossible not to discuss the changes that have taken place in alternative medicine. The Bible says 'Where there is no vision, the people must perish.' Neither of these men could ever be accused of lack of vision – and they also looked at what others had to offer.

I often recall the meeting we once had with an elderly, well-known medical professor, who came to our clinic in the Netherlands. He was slightly eccentric, but had impressive medical qualifications and asked if he could rent the loft of the clinic. There he built a very large contraption and when it was ready we were invited to come and see it. He described the kind of patient he required and then he would show us what the machine was designed for. He selected a suitable patient for the treatment and Dr Vogel and I watched with great interest when we saw him pumping 60 pints of chamomile-scented water through this patient's bowels. This treatment he called 'high-bowel cleansing'. We were amazed when we saw what was eliminated from the bowels.

The bowels take up a large space in the body, and they fill themselves with the body's waste material. When the chemistry is right, elimination to the large intestine takes place unhindered. However, in cases of fermentation or stagnant waste material, problems can occur. After the high-bowel cleansing treatment the patient said that she felt absolutely marvellous, and asked if she would be allowed to have the treatment again. In fact, so did every patient who was given this treatment. This is understandable, because when the bowels are properly emptied, the patient feels much better and more energetic. The importance of complete bowel-cleansing is underrated because people rarely realise how much they benefit if that part of the chemistry is right. Today we have colonic irrigation and enemas, but I was utterly shocked when recently I saw a patient who needed an enema every day and colonic irrigation three times a week. That is a desperate situation because the bowels should perform this task spontaneously. There should be enough stimulation from the friendly bacteria for good bowel function. If that is not the case, then there is cause for concern. This is often seen with irritable bowel syndrome. This condition is an alarm signal that the situation is not right: poor digestion, poor absorption, plus excess stress and worry – and the bowel begins to protest. Do the bowels have anything to do with the three bodies of man? Look at very emotional people, look at the tension we find in the neck and shoulders of such people, where the reflexes of the bowels are present. This may sound unscientific, but it has been proved over the years that if the tension is relieved by way of osteopathy, acupuncture or massage, the bowels can often be coaxed into performing more efficiently.

The real problem is often found around the sigmoid area. The sigmoid is very sensitive, and we can get a small glimpse of what is happening there if we look at the kitchen sink. Sometimes the U-bend under the sink becomes blocked. Luckily, the pipe can be taken apart so that the water and the waste material can be disposed off in a bowl underneath. A similar situation is found in the sigmoid, where waste material can sometimes accumulate in its U-bend, causing fermentation. This is something that *Candida albicans* – which is a yeast parasite – thrives on, which is why it is often found in the sigmoid area. I sometimes remark to my patients that I wish we had the equivalent of a kitchen sink drainage system, so that we could clean out this specific area more easily. Realistically, the only option is to treat the bowels with respect.

Digestion is very important in this process, but even more important is absorption. Good circulation too is as important as correct or efficient elimination. The waste material has a detrimental effect on the blood circulation, which manifests itself through the skin, the lungs and the kidneys.

Colonics and enemas are not always necessary because, after all, the body should be able to eliminate its waste spontaneously. Linoforce, which is a natural remedy based on linseed, can be of great benefit. I have often used this remedy for a practical challenge for students, by asking them to chew a few seeds. If properly masticated, a few seeds result in the production of a large quantity of saliva in the mouth, which in turn facilitates the formation of a motion of the right texture, enabling the smooth and painless elimination of a jellied mass from the body.

The most common complaints I hear from people with irritable bowel syndrome are of irregular motions: sometimes hard, sometimes soft and sometimes as diarrhoea. This is a signal that the diet needs correction.

At any one of the seven clinics where I practise, there are always several patients who complain about this almost fashionable problem of irritable bowel syndrome. It is a chronic intestinal disorder, symptomised by abdominal pain and alteration of the bowel habit, and unfortunately it is often diagnosed as 'cause unknown'. However, we should be aware that it is the stress factor and emotional tension or disharmony that can cause this problem, apart from nutritional deficiencies, and the universal use of refined sugar and flour, chocolate and artificial sweeteners. Sometimes people think that a wholewheat diet may help, but they are mistaken because wheat itself can be a cause of the problem. Extra bran may help, but the first step should be to avoid refined sugars and flours, and artificial additives.

The large intestine, which has to cope with many interferences, sometimes becomes irritated and if conditions are wrong, even a cup of tea or coffee can cause an inflammatory bowel problem. This can lead to diverticular problems or even more serious bowel conditions. Sensitivity to certain foods will also influence any bowel condition. Unfriendly bacteria in the bowels have been shown to be the cause of many conditions where there is a connection between the stomach and the bowels. Bacteria, which are often present in the gelatine-like mucous of the stomach, are sometimes resistant to antibiotics, which are all too often prescribed for this purpose. It is here that a naturopath can often achieve better results than the frequently prescribed antibiotics. The constant discomfort or spasms of pain which characterise irritable bowel syndrome, will not be relieved unless a sensible approach is taken to this problem. The gut behaves erratically, displaying all kinds of symptoms: abdominal tension, bloated stomach, diarrhoea alternating with hard motions, mucus in the stools, headache, loss of appetite, nausea, wind and flatulence, and sometimes even vomiting. It becomes a very complicated problem, but, fortunately, it is not connected with cancer.

Many people find it easier to cope with irritable bowel syndrome once they have learned to relax. I often suggest relaxation and breathing exercises as part of their treatment. A very simple method for releasing tension and stress is to sit quietly, breathing slowly and deeply in through the nose, and out through the mouth, filling the stomach up with air. The entire body then becomes loose and relaxed. Whenever you experience a feeling of acute stress or fear, do these exercises. Take six slow, deep breaths, using the same breathing method as described above, but each time you breathe out, envisage that everything will be all right, that you feel much better . . . and keep doing this exercise. Patients with irritable bowel syndrome have found this simple exercise of great help.

Liquorice and ginger are also very helpful. Ginger has a long history in the treatment of a variety of intestinal ailments. With pregnant women I have often seen how helpful ginger and ginger tea can be for relieving the intestinal spasms that are so often experienced. The herbs peppermint, balm and rosemary are also useful for this purpose. I was amazed how much the insides of man can influence the emotional body. The other day I had to give a lecture and this event, scheduled to take place in a church hall, was over-subscribed. The organiser asked the minister if the venue for the public lecture could be changed to the church itself. Together with the organiser, the minister came to see me and stated that he was prepared to give his permission if I was prepared to speak on herbs mentioned in the Bible. I had very little time to prepare this, yet when I concentrated, I was amazed how frequently some of the above herbs were mentioned in the Bible. In the old translation we read in Psalm 38:8: 'David felt that his bowels were full of a plague and there was nothing wholesome in his flesh.' In more recent translations this verse reads that 'His lungs were filled with burning and there is no soundness in the flesh.' Yet another translation uses the words 'bowels, loins or limbs'. I am sure that the great King David was aware of the holistic principle, possibly intuitively. We now know for sure that if there are problems with the bowels or constipation, poisonous situations occur, infections influence the blood and problems affect the loins or limbs with a stiffness, rheumatism or arthritis.

So we see how essential it is to keep the bowel system in order. Irritable bowel syndrome is only an alarm signal telling us that there is something wrong in that area. The symptoms dictate that we have to look not only at stress and emotions, but that we should consider the three bodies of man holistically.

Constipation actively encourages *Candida albicans* conditions. This yeast parasite loves cheese, mushrooms, sugar, chocolate, wine and any fermented or yeast product, and these food items make the ideal breeding ground for the parasite. In degenerative diseases such as rheumatism, arthritis and cancer, and even conditions such as ME, we often find an active candida situation. It reacts according to the different influences in the bowel, such as the lack of 'friendly' bacteria which is often neglected, until candida flares up with all the possible unpleasant effects mentioned above. Certain foods may cause the candida bacteria to become active, destroying even more of the friendly bacteria. Yet, it is even more important to know that there are foods or remedies which will discourage or destroy these detrimental bacteria, such as the plant devil's claw, from which the remedy *Harpagophytum* is derived, as well as garlic and aloe vera. These remedies are therefore useful in the treatment of stomach disorders, because they encourage the proliferation of friendly bowel bacteria with acidophilus or biodophilus. This knowledge has resulted in the development of an excellent remedy called Acidophilus Extra, which is prescribed to safeguard a favourable balance between the beneficial and putrefactive bacteria in times of stress, travel, illness and changes in the diet; when antibiotics are necessary; and for elderly people, who are prone to such problems. When, in public lectures to a British audience I advise that natural yoghurt should be eaten daily, they look as if I have suggested eating poison. Even worse is the reaction I receive when I recommend drinking a glass of buttermilk every day. Yet these simple steps will be of great benefit in maintaining healthy flora in the bowels.

We cannot ignore problems such as candidiasis, the occurrence of which is very much on the increase. It is sad when people go to the doctor with such a problem only to be told that it is a psychosomatic problem or that they are hypochondriac. This is certainly not the case, because this condition can lead to allergic problems, depression of the immune system, a hormonal imbalance, and may eventually affect the person psychologically. Usually if a patient comes to see me with such a problem, it seems to trigger a sixth sense in me; I am nearly always correct in the diagnosis, even before people have told me about their symptoms. As I have mentioned before, I look, I feel and I listen, but I also smell. The smell from the mouth or the skin can tell us a great deal and when a patient has been taking antibiotics for a long time, that smell can be very penetrating.

The candida bacteria are present in every person. A healthy human gut contains about 3–4 lb of micro-organisms. Candida accounts for less than 5 per cent of the total. One of the reasons why breast-feeding is so beneficial is because breast-milk contains a lot of biodophilus factora, lactopherms, leucocytes and many antibodies. All drug-induced problems can have long-lasting effects. We should make sure that whatever medication is taken, there are no after-effects. I remember an article I read in the *Daily Telegraph* of Monday, 2 June 1991, describing a trial involving ten thousand women in England and Wales for the drug DES – Diethyl stilboestrol. This drug was prescribed between 1940 and 1970, in an attempt to reduce blood poisoning, premature births and stillbirths. Later, this drug was found to be capable of damaging the reproductive system, leading to malignancy and infertility. Among the recorded side-effects of this drug were: structural defects of the vagina and uterus, a high rate of anxiety and depression, abnormalities of the uro-genital system, reduced fertility and problems with pregnancy. Whilst one symptom may be treated, the very drug used against disease can become a threat to health. In the same way, drugs that might destroy bowel bacteria should be avoided where possible. If we look at the rate of surgery in the United Kingdom, there is every reason for concern that drug-induced problems may result in surgery that could have been avoided simply by giving proper consideration to the overall situation.

In the UK some 80,000 people suffer from conditions such as ulcerative colitis or Crohn's disease, covering all age groups, including babies. In these illnesses the digestive tracts – the tracts of the body's system for digesting food – are defective, sometimes developing into ulcerative colitis, where the lining of the colon becomes red and swollen. In the case of Crohn's disease the walls of the intestines or gut may become thicker, so that the food being digested has difficulty in passing through. The cause of this condition still requires much investigation. There is no doubt, however, that the healthier your diet, the less chance there is of such a condition developing. Any outward signs, such as diarrhoea with blood, the passing of mucus, pain in the abdominal area, vomiting or loss of weight, are indications that something is wrong in this part of the body.

There is much we can do to help ourselves overcome non-malignant bowel problems. However, in the case of ulcerative colitis, we have a real problem – and one that must not go untreated as in some cases it can lead to cancer. I repeat that if we study the diet of most people today, it should not come as a surprise that abdominal complaints are so common. The immune system, which is our body's own defence system, requires more consideration than normal. Lymphocytes are like immunological soldiers; they are the antibodies whose task is to destroy invaders. In the lower part of the small bowel, if there is an overlapse, Crohn's disease may be the result. Sometimes this condition may develop as the aftermath of tuberculosis in the family, even some generations back. This may take its toll at a later time. If the problem spreads to the colon there is good reason to fear ulcerative colitis, and I have even seen in cases where there is a nerve insulation problem, and the myelin sheath becomes affected, that the likelihood of multiple sclerosis developing is increased. Of the hundreds of MS patients I have treated, many have been diagnosed as suffering from active candida, or more serious bowel conditions. If the nervous system is involved, the problem may affect the kidneys, and if the muscles are affected a polymyalgic rheumatic condition may develop.

Phytotherapy has some wonderful remedies for the conditions mentioned above. These include melissa, chamomile, valerian, althea and verbascum, all of which can be safely used in the preparation of herbal teas, for beneficial results.

A healthy person usually has a well-functioning stomach and bowel. However, if these organs deteriorate, lungs, muscles, bones and joints may become affected. I have mentioned before that in order to reach a diagnosis, I start by looking, listening and feeling. If we know what to look for, a person's posture gives an immediate indication of their general health. Some years ago I compiled a list of posture deviations or indications for a medical lecture, which I now reproduce below:

Normal posture: Usual position and volume of the stomach and guts, allowing erect, unforced posture, barrel-shaped chest; stomach contents not over-large; sternum and pubic bone aligned.

Salute posture: Caused by heavy stomach and upper abdomen; straightening of the upper back; distension of the sternum; higher position of the midriff; pelvis tilted forwards.

Forward tilted posture: Caused by chronic weakening in the gut and increased stomach contents, causing an essential enlargement of the abdomen; stretching of the upper back and the forward-leaning tendency of the upper body.

Duck position: Because of more intrusive digestive dysfunction greater abdominal space is essential, hence a strong tendency for the pelvis to tilt forwards; widening and raised position of the sternum (sometimes noticeable in a shortening of the neck).

Sagging posture: Found in people with weak muscular structure and digestive dysfunction, causing a rounding in the upper back and a sagging in the abodminal area.

Sower posture: Chronic weakness of the intestines and swellings due to poor waste elimination, causing distended abdomen (reminiscent of a sower carrying a seedbag); because of the sagging weight of the stomach, the upper body tends to over-compensate and tilt backwards.

Drummer position: Symptomatic of major enlargement of the intestinal area due to ineffective elimination and flatulence because of digestive disorders; enlargement and raised position of the sternum (causing the neck to sink between the shoulders); this posture is only possible due to curving of the spine in the upper back and a forward tilt of the pelvis.

We often find that antibiotics are prescribed to control diarrhoea, yet this measure is actually more likely to aggravate the problem. This is a prime example of treating the symptom and not the cause. Diarrhoea occurs as a warning that something is out of sorts in the body, and finding the cause of this must surely be more important than treating the outcome. This is where holistic medicine comes into its own. Very often, instead of taking antibiotics, such complaints may be overcome by a dietary change. Replacing certain nutritional ingredients with rice is helpful, or a naturopathic practitioner will give individual dietary advice – for example a gluten-free diet may be recommended. Diarrhoea can often be controlled with Tormentavena, a herbal preparation with tormentil as its major ingredient. Also an *Acidophilus* supplement may be prescribed in order to maintain the correct balance between the billions of bacteria that colonise our digestive system. Most of these bacteria are harmless and one of the main groups of beneficial bacteria is the *Acidophilus* species. The use of capsules containing *Acidophilus* to support the body's own colonies of friendly bacteria is now an established practice. The supplement Acidophilus Extra is particularly recommended for people who are travelling overseas, taking antibiotics or following a strict yeast-free diet, or for those who wish to maintain good flora balance in the bowel.

I remember my grandmother saying 'Death often makes his house within the bowels.' She would generally recommend the old-fashioned remedy of castor oil for cleansing the bowels, firmly believing that all other factors would then fall into place. In the twenty-five years I have worked in Scotland, I have learned to agree with my grandmother, because I have seen how often death originates in the bowels. In this friendly country many people slowly kill themselves by eating the wrong food, which to my mind is a major contributor to the fact that the rate of bowel cancer is the highest in the world. Alarm signals sent out by the body should never be ignored. Action must be taken when these signals are recognised. Consider applying some of the advice found in this chapter in order to promote healthy bowels as part of the chemistry which will improve the health of the entire body.

12

Healthy Lungs

On the west coast of Scotland, where my clinic is situated, agriculture and dairy farming are common. Historically, there was also a thriving mining community. Some of my other clinics are in more built-up areas, and because of the different locations I come across a variety of medical conditions in my clinics. In London I would be unlikely to come across a case such as the one I was asked to diagnose recently in Scotland, regarding a farmer's wife with breathing problems. It transpired that this lady was suffering from a condition commonly referred to as 'farmer's lung'. This problem is often caused by mouldy hay, and can be accompanied by fever or a chill, but usually also congestion. She was very short of breath and I soon realised that she was one of the worst cases I had ever seen. Furthermore, she was badly constipated. When I enquired further she told me that she had a bowel movement every three to four days, and even then only with great effort. It was important to treat not only the condition that caused her breathing problems: this was probably caused because she helped her husband on the farm, and if there is an inherent weakness, a person is more susceptible to the damage that can be caused by inhaling toxic organic dust from hay, which can result in inflammation of the lungs. In this case not only were her bronchial tubes congested, but so were her bowels. I treated her for both problems and, thankfully, we were successful and her life became very much easier. The lungs can be given a very hard task, which varies according to our environment.

A long time ago, Dr Alfred Vogel and I were working together in our clinic in western Scotland, when one of my patients, who was a local fishmonger, arrived for his appointment. When I had seen him previously I had noticed that his breathing was slightly laboured. I had wanted to enquire further about this, but had restricted this to a hint, to which he had never responded. This time he walked into my consulting rooms while I was having a brief discussion with Dr Vogel about another case, and Dr Vogel immediately asked what was wrong with his breathing. He replied that his breathing was sometimes worse and sometimes better, and that he had a touch of asthma. Dr Vogel, without hesitation, told him it seemed more likely to be an allergy problem. After some allergy tests it was discovered that the fishmonger was not allergic to fish, but to his dog, whom he greatly loved. He admitted that he had suffered for years with his breathing, without knowing the cause. Whenever I meet the fishmonger now, he is always cheerful, and eternally grateful for the effective treatment he received. It was actually quite simple: Dr Vogel told him to take four tablets of Kelpasan every morning with some warm water and some Pollinosan, which is also a highly effective remedy for hay fever allergy. This cleared up his problem once and for all.

The lungs do not like interference; they need to be able to work freely, without hindrance. Allergies, for example to pets, housemite, etc. can cause great difficulty in breathing and the appropriate action should be taken immediately. If this problem is allowed to linger, it is likely to get worse, rather than better. In today's society these problems occur more and more frequently. When I wrote my book *Air – The Breath of Life*, little did I realise that it would appear on the market in the midst of major concerns about the phenomenal increase in asthma and bronchitis, largely caused by air pollution.

The issue of pollution, both general and specific, is a great cause for concern. Some people appear to be able to adapt, but others suffer badly as the result of environmental changes. Over a lengthy period of time precisely co-ordinated metabolic reactions and living organisms incorporate air, water and food into themselves. Accidental spills of herbicides, pesticides and artificial fertilisers, and pollution from the air have caused the respiratory system great problems. In *The Guardian* of 4 July 1994 I read that the increase of asthma is keeping pace with the increase in pollution. The growing incidence of illness linked to air pollution was highlighted in a report showing a five-fold increase in families requesting financial help for children with asthma and severe skin complaints. The article recounted how following a weekend of dangerously high air pollution a warning had been given by a consultant in respiratory medicine at a London hospital that not enough beds were available to cope with the extra asthma cases caused by heatwave smog. The Chief Executive of the National Asthma Campaign had commented that air pollution and the whole environment are key areas of research into asthma, which is the only chronic controllable illness on the increase in the western world. The weekend air pollution, with ozone levels reaching 95 parts per billion (ppb), against the 70 ppb recommended by the World

Health Organisation, had highlighted the risks. The report went on to say that asthma costs the nation about £1m per annum, and that traffic pollution was an avoidable trigger. This represents a very sad situation, and from my own research into asthma for my book on that subject I quickly became only too aware of the growing extent of this problem. We must pay attention to the immune system and work at keeping it as effective as possible, only then may it be possible to withstand the pollutive factors.

Many allergies are the result of a lowered immune system. Pollution, whether it be present in the air, water or food, has a detrimental effect on our lungs. Breathing disorders are the order of the day. My fishmonger was fortunate that his condition could be kept under control and that he can still keep his dog. We must never sit back and just learn to live with the situation; we must fight this problem, and by doing so we will achieve a better quality of life. In another article which appeared in *The Guardian* on 7 July 1994, I read that the record traffic pollution level was said to have led to a 10 per cent rise in the death rate in London. Government health officials admitted that this figure, unfortunately, was correct. In a Canadian paper I also read that more than a hundred sick workers at the Camphill Medical Centre were still struggling on a daily basis to resolve several issues surrounding their breathing difficulties and specific lung problems. Although I have only quoted a few isolated examples here, many similar reports regularly appear in our newspapers, certainly too many to quote, but they all spell problems.

The immune system is highly complex and despite our lack of under-standing of the endocrine system, we know that there is a close connection between the two; in other words, the well-being of the endocrine system will determine the effectiveness of the immune system. The healthier our lifestyle and the more outdoor exercise we take, the better it is for our general health. It is important to swim, walk and cycle as much as we can, and in this way support the functioning of our lungs. Breathing exercises are all well and good, but if they are taken in the fresh air, they will be doubly beneficial. The long-standing principle of rest, light, air and sunshine is still valid.

I had several cousins who suffered from lung disease, and in the early years after the Second World War, they were sent to Arosa in Switzerland, as was customary at that time. I remember looking at the lovely photographs they showed on their return, among them one from the front entrance of the sanatorium, where the words were displayed: 'Lift your eyes unto the hills, whence cometh your health.' They thrived on the fresh and thinner air in the high altitude of the Swiss Alps. They came back feeling refreshed and healthy, but once they had spent some time in the damp and industrial atmosphere in the Netherlands, their health soon deteriorated again. Unfortunately, today even in Arosa in Switzerland the air is not what it used to be. Air pollution affects us everywhere. We have to arm ourselves, and building up our immune system is the most effective way to achieve this. The forces of healing can only work if we give them a fair chance.

To better understand the immune system, I will again refer to the endocrine system. Activation of the T-lymphocytes, which produce lymphokines and hormone-like ACTH, will enhance the process that feeds back to the brain and informs the body's immune system. The traffic between the brain and the immune system is two-way. The endorphins released by the pituitary gland will affect different parts of the body. They not only feed back to the brain, but the brain endorphins influence the immune cells. The possible peripheral sites of action will have an effect on the nerves, vascular system, heart, lungs and other tracts. This system shows that the three bodies – physical, mental and emotional – should be in harmony. It is not uncommon in people with lung problems for a bout of breathing difficulties to be triggered by an emotional upset. Such an attack can be relieved by acupuncture, osteopathy or chiropractic treatment, or by simple hot- and cold-water treatments. Each case should be dealt with individually. Breathing should be rhythmic; tension and relaxation are two very closely related factors in people with lung problems. It is often a give and take situation. The more we try to relax ourselves, to free ourselves to breathe in air, the easier it will be.

Pollution will stand in our way, but we are not going to accept that as an excuse and by swimming, walking, cycling and breathing correctly, we can try to help the immune system, or let us call it the brain system, to overcome such problems. I often see asthmatic or bronchial people who ignore their condition and want to do too much. It is better that they accept the situation and concentrate on simple ways to alleviate their condition by taking some practical steps. They should watch their diet, because dairy foods, such as milk, cheese, butter and cream all contain mucus-forming agents, which congest the lungs. Emotionally they must try to come to terms with the limitations of their situation.

Calcium and some supplementary vitamins should be taken to compensate for deficiencies. I can wholeheartedly recommend Urticalcin, a combination of calcium and nettle extract, for any lung or respiratory related problems: twice a day, five tablets. A very good vitamin combination, such as Health Insurance Plus, and garlic capsules are also beneficial for people with breathing problems. I have twice had pneumonia, and even though I recovered quickly, I needed help to do so. I meditated and tried to relax. I prayed to get better, and this certainly helped to ease the situation. During the dreadful coughing bouts I experienced, I tried not to fight it. I took Echinaforce and garlic capsules to speed up my recovery. When my brother went down with pleurisy, in her old-fashioned way, my mother applied hot- and cold-water compresses to reduce the inflammation of the pleura, and control the respiritory problems and his coughing.

Not even a cough should be ignored, as it is an indication that the immune system is struggling to stay in control, and an untreated cough can lead to more serious respiratory problems. These are the times to take extra vitamin C, when up to 2 grammes daily may be taken. As the body is unable to manufacture this vitamin, an adequate daily intake is necessary, and if the diet does not supply this nutrient in sufficient quantity, it will be essential to take a supplement.

Vitamin C has such marvellous and diverse qualities:

- It is involved in cell and tissue repair.
- It is involved in the conversion of proline to hydroxyproline and is therefore essential in collagen maintenance in skin, bones and teeth.
- It is required for the activity of leucocytes, immunoglobins and natural antibodies.
- It protects vitamins A and E against damage.
- It helps to maintain normal blood cholesterol levels.
- It has antioxidant properties.
- It is involved in the formation of corticosteroid hormones in the adrenal gland.

When taken together with a high dose of Echinaforce – at such times as much as thirty drops may be taken three times daily – most common coughs will disappear, and if this is not the case then please see your medical practitioner, because the cause for this lingering cough should be investigated. A wheeze may have disturbed the harmony in the body, and the lung function may be impaired as a consequence. Simple remedies such as pine kernels may be used. When we open a pine kernel a strong expectorant smell is released, which helps to unblock the respiratory organs. That is why Dr Vogel chose the pine kernel as the main ingredient, together with honey, in Santasapina, which is a very effective herbal cough syrup.

In the case of obstruction in the bronchi caused by asthma, kelp, Asthma drops, supplementary garlic and/or a calcium supplement, will be of help. Bronchosan is a combination remedy specifically designed with the bronchitis patient in mind. Together with a hot lemon and honey drink, Bronchosan is an excellent remedy for respiratory problems. I recently recommended this remedy during a radio broadcast in Ireland, and in the same context I mentioned the old-fashioned remedy Irish Moss. The radio station received numerous phone calls after the broadcast, which confirmed my belief that people are interested in ways to help themselves, if only they are shown the way. Even irreversible bronchial problems can be relieved, such as bronchiectasis, or a 'miner's lung', which I have come across all too often in the south-west of Scotland.

For several generations my father's family was involved in the tobacco industry, and as a result several of my relatives developed lung disease. I am convinced that, one way or another, most of these problems were related to tobacco. As a youngster I remember seeing rows of men in the factory, rolling cigars, and chewing away on the off-cuts. At one time, the rate of tuberculosis among the factory workers became so high that something had to be done about it. I also remember the poverty among the factory workers, and the men having to work extremely hard to achieve their daily quota of cigars. It is a frightening thought that luxury items such as tobacco and alcohol have extracted their toll, first on the health of the people involved in the production and second on the health of the users. These non-essential, self-indulgent stimulants disturb the three bodies of man. We should bear in mind, however, that harmony is still present in nature, even though man constantly tries to disturb it. Although the air may be polluted, the force of nature will help to restore imbalances, and with common sense it will help to remedy the balance in man's breathing.

13

Healthy Bones

As an osteopath with more than thirty-five years experience, I have seen thousands of patients with skeletal problems. The reason why I have purposely chosen to follow the chapter on respiratory and asthmatic problems with this subject, is because one should always view the body holistically, bearing in mind the three bodies of man – the physical, the mental and the emotional bodies.

I will never forget the day I learned that I had lost one of my dearest friends. We had been friends for many years, and had a very honest relationship, being able to communicate freely on all kinds of topics. She had certainly had her problems, and she was a very emotional person with very deep feelings. For a long time she had been asthmatic, and her condition had been strongly affected by some of the emotional changes and tensions she experienced in her life. However, the way she died was extremely hard to accept. Her husband, a very able general practitioner and a close friend of my wife and I, had taken good care of her and had kept her going so that her asthmatic condition did not greatly interfere in her life. She had experienced a lot of sadness and distress, which had taken its toll of her immune system. Late one afternoon she was cycling to a local shop when she was hit by a car and knocked off her bike. She was taken to hospital, and it seemed that she had only suffered minor concussion. Her asthmatic problem, however, became worse, and in the hospital it was concluded that this was because of the shock of the accident. X-rays were taken of her neck, but there did not appear to be a problem. Unfortunately, no one thought to take X-rays of her back, and this is where the problem started. Her asthmatic problem deteriorated and she became more congested. One evening, when her husband came to visit her in the hospital, he was stopped by the ward sister who informed him that she was not fit enough to receive visitors. When he told the sister that he was not only her husband but also a doctor, she asked him to wait. The specialist came immediately and told him that, sadly, his wife had died five minutes previously. She had been a young woman, and on closer examination it was concluded that she could have been saved if her spine had been X-rayed, because it would have become clear that a spinal deviation had caused her breathing to deteriorate, ending disastrously in her untimely death.

Every disc or vertebra in the spine has a function, and in this case the third, fourth and fifth dorsal or thoracic vertebra with the associated ribs were seen to be exerting severe pressure. Because of that, my friend, this charming young woman, had not been able to breathe properly. It was this unhappy event that influenced my decision to follow the chapter on asthma with a chapter on bones and skeletal structure.

In my book *Back and Neck Problems* I have explained the different problems that can occur, from the point of view of an osteopath. Even if bones are misaligned or compressed, providing care is taken, they may continue to function satisfactorily. Every bone in the body must receive care and nutrition. Exercise is as necessary to the bones as is correct nutrition. There is no need for problems such as osteoporosis or misalignment to occur, if proper care is taken. People usually think that our bones move voluntarily, but in fact it is the muscles that move the bones, and you will find more information on this aspect of the skeleton in the next chapter. Bones are built from tissue, and in these bone cells there is constant degeneration and regeneration. Although our bones may look strong they can be very brittle, and the skeletal condition is highly dependent on age and nutrition.

Organic components, which are needed to form the cell tisssue of the bone, are built up from calcium salts, phosphates, chlorides, fluorides and citrates, and the proportion in which they are present is a decisive factor in the flexibility of the bones. The cell tisssue between the bones is called ossein, and this determines the elasticity. It can be likened to a gelatinous mass that keeps the bone flexible. The outside of the bone is quite hard and compact, whilst the inside is more like a sponge in structure, as can be clearly observed when looking at a bone through a microscope. The living tissue in the bones, as in all parts in the body, is dependent on oxygen. The periosteum, which is a tough membrane covering the bones, contains nerves and small veins, which in the ribs and the breast bone is formed by different blood cells. The osteons form a central channel, known as the 'Channel of Havers'. Around the bone we see highly concentrated bone lamellae, and the structural types are clearly understood to be separate. The bone cells, or osteocytes, which are part of the lamellae, are also called canaliculi. These little channels, sometimes referred to as the 'Channels of Volkmann', form a radiant connection between the bone cells within the osteon. The bone cells that have become calcified because of poor nutrition can be eliminated. The outer ends of the bones, or the bone beams, are called the trabeculae. Every bone beam has an elastic organism. The activity of the bone cells is related to the pressure which is placed on the bone, which is why if a bone breaks, it is very important to relieve the pressure to encourage healing. In such cases, where the bone is still growing, as in young people, this will help the healing process, whereas a bone fracture in elderly people will take longer to mend.

Hormones play a significant role in the growth of bones, as do vitamin D and calcium, and the amount of calcium in the blood needs to be carefully regulated. I have seen many problems caused by the incorrect use of nutritional supplements and minerals.

I have already mentioned that there is constant degeneration and regeneration occurring within the bones. There are bone-formers, also called osteoblasts, and bone-eaters, called osteoclasts. This subject leads us to consideration of the often serious condition of osteoporosis. This is an ever-increasing problem, closely related to nutrition, lifestyle, lack of exercise and drug use. Combined, these factors determine the level of degeneration within the bones, possibly resulting in an osteoporotic condition. On occasions, when I have been asked to treat patients with manipulation, I have had to refuse such treatment because the bones have become too brittle as a result of osteoporosis and manipulation would be dangerous.

Nowadays, women are often advised to take HRT – Hormone Replacement Therapy. This is claimed to cure or prevent osteoporotic conditions, but I have my doubts. Especially in the USA women appear to feel that when they turn fifty, life has little left to offer. They feel that they are no longer attractive to the opposite sex, and they believe that by taking HRT their skin will retain its elasticity and remain youthful and that they will also safeguard themselves against osteoporosis. If this was true in every case, it would be fine, and if I believe there is no other option than recommending HRT, then I will advise my patient to be extremely careful. We still have a lot to learn about the endocrine system and the hormonal system, and we do not yet know for certain how these systems will react to a long-term hormonal supplement. I become suspicious when, as a naturopath, I have had to treat women who take HRT for phlebitis, thrombosis and in some cases breast cancer. We cannot be too careful with such supplements.

Certainly, the bones of elderly people become more brittle, and infections such as periostitis, arthritis, or even osteomyelitis, can occur, because the bones can be attacked by a number of underlying causes. If the bones become soft and lose their strength, there are ways in which this can be overcome. Dr Vogel, quite a few years ago now, while sitting in his study noticed some stinging nettles growing in a flower bed. He pondered on these and eventually decided that if the stinging nettles were mixed with a calcium supplement, this would help the absorption of calcium in the body. The eventual outcome of his experiments was the wonderful remedy Urticalcin, which has proved to be of tremendous value in cases of bone degeneration. OsteoPrime, which is a combination of specific vitamins, minerals and trace elements, has also proved to be a great ally for people with similar bone degenerative conditions.

Bone is more than just a collection of calcium crystals; it is active, living tissue. Healthy bones need a variety of nutrients to preserve an adequate mineral mass, to strengthen their supporting structures, and to promote their repair functions. Obviously, calcium is important – more than 99 per cent of the body's calcium is found in the bones and teeth. But calcium alone is not enough: the body needs vitamin D to utilise the calcium together with phosphorus for building strong bones and teeth. Magnesium activates enzymes that help form new calcium crystals. Vitamin K aids the production of osteocalcin, the supporting structure on which calcium crystallises in the bone. Manganese is needed for bone mineralisation and connective tissue synthesis. Studies also show that zinc, strontium, vitamin B_6, vitamin C, silicon, copper and boron are all instrumental in the formation of the connective structures in bone.

From the moment that primitive man started to walk upright, his skeleton underwent an evolutionary transformation. Certain bones took on a new role and as a result started to move in a different manner. The muscles that move the bones had to adjust in order to support an upright posture. Basically, the more bones we move, the better, otherwise problems of bone deviation can occur. These include not only osteoporosis, but also osteomalacia, or pseudo-fractures, or problems like Paget's disease and many more. Over the years we have learned how to overcome or compensate for such problems and even in cases of osteomyelitis, where there is infection in the bone, there are many effective alternative methods that can be applied. Bacteria invading the bone, via the blood, can lead to bone disease. Therefore proper bone nutrition, requiring a healthy diet, is vital. I am always sorry when I hear that doctors or practitioners do not take the opportunity to make this sufficiently clear to their patients. At every lecture I emphasise that if nutrition is neglected serious health problems may develop as the years go by. A basically healthy diet and some supplementary vitamins, minerals and trace elements are the foundations of a healthy bone structure.

Remember that pain is never felt within the bone, it is always in the tissue. Although I have practised manipulation on many patients, the power in the hands, if correctly used on certain pressure points, can encourage the body to cure itself. I learned much in this field from my tutor Dr Leonard Allan, who in turn gives credit to his friend George Ivan Carter. The method of letting the body's own energy do the work is a real pleasure to watch and study. There is no need for any force. In the Far East I once watched a slipped disc being successfully treated with pressure no more than that exerted by the thumb. The simple formula used by practitioners is to hold the opposite: if one bone or area has to be dropped to an energy pool, this is to be held from underneath; the opposite side, usually touched by the thumb or fingers from the upper side, allows the flow of body energy from the practitioner to aid the patient. This process is called bone symmetry.

Unfortunately, the stresses of life have a negative effect on both the nervous system and the blood circulatory system. The muscles and bones both register this stress, but it is given little attention. If people would only realise the misery and distress that can be caused by the mastoid bone and the neck being out of position. I see it on a regular basis, virtually daily, and I am able to recognise it at first glance. When examining a patient, I look immediately to see if the neck is straight and if the left and right ear are in balance. If not, I use a simple bone symmetry treatment, or a mild soft-tissue manipulation. So many mistakes are made by hard and fixed manipulation, especially on the third cervical vertebra, which is often out of alignment. This should always be handled carefully to avoid causing permanent damage, as that single vertebra controls the entire sympathetic nervous system.

The neck can become sore and stiff, sometimes accompanied with pain, and if out of alignment, it interferes with the teeth, restricting the blood circulation and flow of nerve energy. Such a disalignment may also be the underlying cause of a bone infection. Holistically, the bowels often affect the top of the nerve, especially if there is a build-up of wind and flatulence. The first step in the treatment of this problem is to check the alignment of the neck and shoulders. A crooked neck, or shoulders that are out of alignment, will invariably affect the internal organs.

The shoulder blades are responsible for the condition of the neck. If the right shoulder is lower and appears to be longer than the left shoulder, you will find the left shoulder blade to be higher than the right one. When examining the back of the shoulder, you will find a large solid lump. The right shoulder blade will have moved down and there will be very little tension, if any, above the shoulder blades. The right shoulder blade will crowd the spine out of position to the left, or closer to the left shoulder blade. This causes the seventh cervical, or the large bone on the back of the neck, to move to the left also. The cervical region, or neck bones, will have moved to the right and caused the atlas or top bone of the neck to twist out of position. When closely examining the front of the neck, we often find that the right side of the neck seems to be a trifle larger and firmer. Here is the starting point of trouble with the eyes, ears, nose and mouth, and migraine headaches. The neck will become prominent or very full on the left side, while on the right side a depression will be noticed that will interfere with the breathing. Such cases have been known to be connected to tuberculosis of the lungs.

The reverse condition indicates a susceptibility to asthma. It will be obvious to anyone who thinks about it that when standing with the left shoulder lowered, the spine will move to a different position. When the left shoulder is raised, the opposite shoulder drops. Movement of the spine from one position to another may cause the ligaments under the higher shoulder to become rigid inside the body, and the opposite side becomes so relaxed that it forces the internal organs to move out of place and become congested. If any disturbance is present, especially in the heart area, different parts of the body begin to move out of place. A twist in the neck or disalignment of the shoulders may interfere with the entire nervous system. Once a disturbance has reached the autonomous nervous system then the whole body develops some peculiar and dangerous symptoms which are generally misdiagnosed as a disease. Complications produced by any disturbance in the energy field have far-reaching implications. They can affect the glandular or endocrine system. Observing the human frame always presents a clear picture of the human being who owns that frame. Blood toxins can be eliminated by means of observation and the application of bone symmetry methods. In a roundabout way, disturbance of the human frame affects the lymphatic drainage, which can be even more important than the blood flow.

The lymphatics are greater in number than the arteries and veins, and have connections with all parts of the internal organs. They inhabit the skin of the body, face and scalp and have strong influence on the thyroid gland. They carry sensory action to all parts of the body and any sense, good or bad, is affected by the condition of the lymph. The action and movement of any part of the neck and hands are influenced by the lymph.

If the lymph becomes thick and sluggish it gradually slows down the action of the blood as the gland supplies lymph to the red blood. The more active the lymph becomes the more quickly the body will move. The lymphatic system consists of a complex network of connecting vessels which conduct the lymph from the various organs and tissues of the body to the large veins of the neck, connecting with the jugular veins and veins of less importance, where the lymph is poured into the bloodstream. In this system of connecting vessels there are many lymph glands or nodes. These little nodes, or sacs, which act as filters separating one substance from another, resemble buttons on a string and are placed at different distances apart. By using our fingers, we can actually feel the relation between the components of the lymphatic group, which carries the sense of vibration of our body. All that is necessary is to trace the lymphatics and to draw the finger of the right hand along the corresponding finger on the opposite hand, and we will get a sensation of touch.

In the field of bone symmetry there is much that can be done. A cranial osteopath can correct bones of the skull that have moved out of position. I'll take the jaw bone as an example. If the left side of the skull is low, the right side will be forced out of position. This forces the teeth on the left side of the mouth to close much more firmly than on the right side, and in this case we are inclined to chew our food on the left side of the mouth only. By doing this we keep the pressure of the teeth on the right side, which will impede nerve action and the circulation of blood to both the upper and lower teeth on that side of the face. In many cases this is the cause of ulcers on the gums, toothache and gingivitis, for which the remedy Co-Enzyme Q10 can provide great relief. A condition like this can also cause the sinus or facial bone to twist out of shape and, what is worse, the jaw bone or the TM joint moves and this can cause serious facial neuralgia. Even sciatica can be caused by a misaligned jaw or pressure on the TM joint or hyoid bone. I have seen the most awful cases in my time and thankfully I have been able to develop, with the help of a Dutch colleague, a special manipulation technique to control these misaligned jaw bones and put them back into place.

If we look closely at the bones of the face, one eye might appear to be lower than the other. This is an indication that the facial bones are out of position. Then the frontal or forehead bone will show the same signs, thus moving the bone of the forehead down on the left side, causing the left eye to be lower. As the left side of the frontal part of the skull moves downward, it naturally causes the back of the skull on the same side to move upwards. This will interfere with the position of the mastoid gland, bringing unnatural pressure to bear on the medulla and interfering with the sight and hearing as it causes the mastoid bone to rise, corresponding with the back of the skull. This movement will prevent the head from being in a straight position on the atlas, impinging the nerves of the spine, and causing a lack of energy in the brain, eyes, ears, nose and throat. Thus, to a certain extent, the circulation is cut off to the different parts of the head and face. Osteopathic or chiropractic treatment may then be necessary, but I should stress that this should only be undertaken by a fully qualified professional. Bone symmetry exercises can also be done by the patient, and I have described some of these exercises in my book *Body Energy*. Once again, to keep these bones healthy and fit, a wholesome diet providing correct nutrition is essential.

The mastoid bone is located just behind the ears along the base of the skull, between the temporal and the occipital bones. Misalignment of the mastoid bone cannot only interfere with our hearing, it can also affect our balance. The mastoid bone is also prone to infections, and we should not underestimate the seriousness of the problems that can ensue.

It is sometimes possible to locate the cause of a problem simply by passing the palm of the hand over the body. When we come to a cold spot, the organ beneath the cold spot needs attention. It may be that the gall bladder is impaired, or the gall duct. If we can find the cold spot for any organ, for example the pancreas, or the spleen, on the opposite side of the body, on the left side just at the bottom of the ribs, then put your right hand on the ribs when these particular spots are treated. So many parts of the body have a direct connection with the brain and a correct connection between these three bodies of man is important. The cynic will probably think that this is nonsense, but the cynic will also claim to know the price of everything, and value of nothing. There is great simplicity in these treatments.

A simple treatment method for misalignment of the mastoid bone is to place the thumbs on the mastoid and hold them there. In the upper scapula or shoulder blade, a whole range of different neck and back problems can be balanced by placing the thumb on the relative bone. The same goes for aligning the knees: hold the thumbs firmly on the side of both knees. For the upper jaw, the correct location is just above the ears. For the sinuses, the location is just above the bridge of the nose, between the eyes. To align the nostrils, press firmly next to the nostrils. There are many methods that can be used for simple bone symmetry. It is a wonderful part of osteopathy which enables us to restore harmony in the three bodies by physical touch.

Location of spinal nerve centres for polarity therapy

Visceral centres in the spine

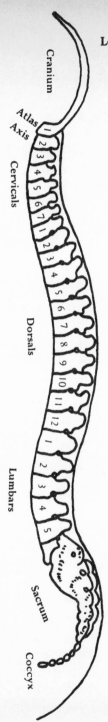

Structures in the head – 2nd and 3rd dorsals and the 7 upper cervicals.

Larynx and thyroid gland – 3rd dorsals and cervical area.

Bronchi – 3rd and 4th dorsals with associated ribs.

Heart – 4th and 5th dorsals with associated ribs.

Lungs – 3rd, 4th and 5th dorsals with associated ribs.

Diaphragm – 4th and 5th cervicals.

Stomach – 5th to 8th dorsals.

Small intestines, first portion – 8th and 9th dorsals.

Small intestines, last portion – 9th to 12th dorsals.

Liver – 8th and 9th dorsals.

Gall bladder – 10th dorsal. Also rib on right side.

Kidney – 11th and 12th dorsals.

Appendix – 12th dorsal. Also 12th rib on right side.

Ovaries and testes – 2nd lumbar.

Uterus – 2nd and 5th lumbar (Hypogastric plexus).

Sciatica – 11th and 12th dorsals. 1st, 2nd and 3rd lumbar.

Bladder – 5th lumbar.

Haemorrhoids – coccyx.

Spastic sphincter – Anti-coccyx.

Place right hand or middle finger on visceral centre as indicated and left hand over part to be treated. Hold for one or two minutes.

125

Let's look at a very common complaint – whiplash injury. A whiplash is in effect an invisible handicap. It can occur as the result of an emergency stop in a car, or a drastic movement of the neck, or any kind of accident. The damage can be very slight and when an X-ray is taken this hairline crack is often overlooked. Dizziness, headaches, neck pain, lapses of concentration, memory loss and insomnia are all symptoms that may result from a whiplash. Some whiplash patients can overcome their problems quickly if given the correct treatment but, unfortunately, all too often these injuries go unnoticed and so remain untreated. Sometimes it is even suggested that there is something mentally wrong with the patient. It is true that the three bodies of man are involved – mentally, physically and emotionally – and although the physical body is hurt the emotional effect cannot be ignored either. Yet I always feel sorry for patients who have been told that they have a mental problem, or that they are hypochondriacs, for their physical symptoms are all too real. Nevertheless, after correct treatment for a whiplash condition they will soon be back to normal. Some of the remedies I tend to prescribe for whiplash are Galeopsis or Araniforce, a tissue-healing remedy, together with Urticalcin. I might also apply some gentle manipulation.

For all healing in the body relaxation is necessary. Stress will influence the mental, physical and emotional bodies, particularly the glands, organs and muscles, often causing an imbalance of the glandular and nervous systems. The ability of the body to cope with stress effectively is fundamental to good health. By correcting vertebral supplications and fixations and by balancing the body in other ways, the chiropractor and the osteopath will relieve major stresses, which will help the bones and muscles to operate efficiently. Every disc has a function. In the cervical spine discs C1, C2 and C3 look after the blood supply to the head, scalp, inner and middle ear, eyes, sinuses and forehead. When dizziness and problems of tinnitus and vertigo are experienced, we often find that the blood supply to the brain is restricted in these upper three discs. Discs C4 and C5 will look after the nose, lips, mouth, Eustachian tubes, vocal chords, neck, glands and the diaphragm. Problems in these areas may be alleviated by releasing these bones using either soft-tissue manipulation or bone symmetry. Discs C6 and C7 control the neck muscles, shoulders, arms and hands. Then, going to the thoracic or dorsal spine discs T1, T2 and T3 control the heart, lungs, trachea, oesophagus and bronchi, whilst T4 and T5 control the gall bladder and the liver. Discs T6 through to T9 control the stomach, pancreas, spleen, adrenals and the abdominal muscles, while T10, T11 and T12 control the kidneys, the small intestine, the ovaries and the uterus. In the lumbar spine discs L1, L2 and L3 control the large intestine, the bladder and knee problems. I have been asked on countless occasions to treat the knees where no more was needed than some adjustment to the spinal discs. Discs L4 and L5 control the prostate gland, lower hip, back, buttocks, sciatic nerve, legs and feet. A seriously debilitating condition such as sciatica can often be relieved when gentle pressure is applied to L4 and L5.

I am called upon to treat many patients with a so-called slipped disc, or a prolapse of the intervetebral disc. They think they can be helped on the spot by having the disc clicked back in place. Often, they even tell me that they heard it 'go'. It is not like that at all, and the best way to explain this injury is to think of the disc as a cream chocolate. If the disc is injured, it is as though the cream inside the chocolate has been squashed, and when the cream flows out of the chocolate, as it were onto the spinal nerve, it causes inflammation. It usually takes a little time for this condition to be completely overcome. The irritation caused if the discs are not correctly aligned can be the cause of very real pain. Responsible treatment is essential, so as to avoid the risk of serious problems such as ankylosing spondilitis, other spondilitic conditions and arthritic conditions and problems where the spine directs certain parts of the body, either positively or negatively.

Lower-back pain is an ever-growing problem, and is often caused by lack of regular exercise, or the wrong posture when lifting something heavy. It is possible that many patients who have been the victim of a laminectomy could well have been treated without the need for surgery. If a laminectomy is really the only way out then I have no objection provided this is considered only as a last resort, but all too often I fear that other methods have not been given a proper chance. I was delighted when a well-known surgeon spent a day working alongside me at my clinic. At the end of the day he said that it was time to review our anatomy. He was sorry that he had performed so many back operations, having realised that many of them were probably unnecessary, because the patients could have been helped by some other form of treatment, such as acupuncture or osteopathy, proper nutrition and herbal medicine. Certainly, disc degeneration does lead to a loss of disc height, as disc material is lost and consequently an instability of the posterior joints develops. Sometimes this has led to a degree of supplication of the vertebral segments. However, in lumbar disc degeneration, which is sometimes part of the ageing process, positive steps can be taken to relieve the degeneration or chronic inflammation.

The psychological aspect of lower back pain also needs to be taken into consideration and this is where a holistic approach is important, i.e. the relation between mind, body and soul. I do not believe that imbalances always have a physical cause. I have seen the stresses and tensions which especially can settle in the neck. If tension or stress is apparent, for instance, in the third cervical disc, it often corresponds with the ninth dorsal disc. This may cause problems elsewhere in the body. That particular disc usually corresponds with the third and fourth lumbar disc, which can cause circulation problems. Unbalanced tensions can cause the bones to assume an incorrect position, leading to more strain, than would be the case if the level of tension were normal. Moreover, the weakened part of the ligaments permits a motion in the direction of a possible lesion.

However, it is not my purpose in this book to write about an osteopathic approach to health. Primarily, my aim is to show that the three bodies of man all need to be taken into consideration when treating any health problem. Therefore in describing the method known as body symmetry I have tried to explain briefly what we can do with our own hands, and how to balance our bones and muscles. We have grown away from our initial creation, because our vertebrae are not really constructed for upright posture. Countless generations ago we evolved to stand on our hind limbs, thus enabling us to use the hands freely and develop the brain. The way we move now requires the entire spine to carry tremendous tension. The lumbar spine carries the full body weight and, like the cervical spine, is subject to tension and nerves. The sensation of pain which develops in the brain is subject to the moods of the patient. Some pains persist until the cause is removed, and especially with chronic depression it is common for chronic lumbago to be a side-effect. This is not to say that it is just a psychological problem; sometimes even the opposite is true. Prevention is better than cure, and therefore physical and mental exercise and relaxation should become part of our daily routine.

It seems that thirteen million working hours are lost each year as a result of back conditions. These can have a variety of causes: accidents, sport injuries, incorrect lifting, poor posture when seated – all exerting pressure to the five bones comprising the lumbar spine. It is most frequently compression, due to poor nutrition, that changes the structure of the disc. The nucleus pulposis, which is a colourless, transparent jelly, and the buffer between the discs, is in some cases almost worn away completely. The way we live, move and exercise is reflected in the condition of the bones.

The thoracic bones differ from the lumbar bones. The bodies of the vertebrae – which are held by the same long bands which extend up to the front and the back bones, where each vertebral body is separated and cushioned from the adjacent discs – are all supposed to work in harmony. The spinal cord extends from the base of the brain to the sacrum. The entire system has to work perfectly, without any interference, and although it is often taken for granted we should do all that lies within our power to help this mechanism in every way we can.

I was surprised to learn that in 800 BC, the ancient Greeks were aware of the minor vibrations that could cause disharmony in the spine. Even Louis Pasteur, in 1862, saw the problems in the magnetic field as positive and negative, and regarded the spine as subject to man's positive and negative energies. Biomagnetic fields within and immediately around the body are very weak compared to the magnetic fields of the earth. It is widely accepted that electric currents move within and through the body. If used correctly, small electric currents can be used to benefit health. This is clearly proven by electro-acupuncture and transcutaneous nerve stimulation. The tremendous relief experienced by people following treatment with electro-acupuncture proves without doubt that even small vibrations can be positively directed if used in the right circumstances. Historically, magnetic therapy has been used by many cultures. Many centuries ago it was used in ancient Egypt and by Greek physicians like Hippocrates and Galen, and in the Middle Ages by Paracelsus. These well-known physicians all found magnetic therapy beneficial. In magnetic therapy, by using the north pole and the south pole to achieve balance, we can bring things back into harmony. These types of therapy can be performed safely and without side-effects.

I am pleased that over the years we have been able to successfully treat bone deformities using osteopathy and acupuncture, together with natural remedies. It is remarkable to see how small bone deformities can be rectified with the help of cranial osteopathy. Such conditions may have been caused by a forceps delivery, for example, and with a multi-disciplinary programme we are often able to restore balance. It is also important to balance the bone structure, and this can be achieved by some of the techniques mentioned above. Of course, it should be remembered that the bones and muscles work closely together.

I remember a lady patient who I treated at my clinic in Ireland. She had contracted osteomyelitis, and was, as she put it, 'completely beyond repair'. Surgery was out of the question under the circumstances. She then purposefully followed a naturopathic programme, taking Petasan, Echinaforce and Urticalcin, followed by acupuncture and soft-tissue manipulation. Whenever I see her now she always brings a smile to my face.

Healthy bones contribute to a healthy life, because the condition of the bones greatly influences the all-over picture of health. Think about how the harmony among bones, muscles and joints keeps the body together – and this is where the skills of a qualified osteopath or chiropractor can play such a big part.

14

Healthy Joints

The first patient I saw after I finished dictating the chapter on healthy bones was a middle-aged lady, the wife of a local retailer. She told me that she helped her husband in his business and often stepped in to serve behind the counter in their shop. She had always been in good health, but lately she had noticed that her legs were swelling. This upset her because the nature of her work required that she spent most of the day on her feet. She had been told by her doctor that the swelling was due to a lymphatic problem and that there was very little he could do. She just had to take things a bit easier. So here she was, asking if there was anything to be done. When I examined her I was surprised to see that one leg was much more swollen than the other. I noticed her varicose veins, and also that her feet were cold. In response to my questions I learned that ever since the menopause she had begun to experience digestion problems and constipation, and these had probably been the cause of her varicose veins and haemorrhoids. However, this was not the whole picture. She also had circulatory problems, but I was particularly concerned by the fact that one of her ankles was considerably more swollen than the other and I asked her if this ankle was particularly sensitive. When I tested this joint I realised that there was very little movement, and also that it caused her considerable discomfort. I immediately noticed that the foot had become flattened and subsequently found that her cuboid bone was out of place. The cuboid bone in the foot, although small, is a very important bone and, unfortunately, in the case of many arthritic and rheumatic patients this bone is out of place. So it was with this lady and in her case the flexibility of the ankle was very poor. I told her that unless I treated the ankle first I would not be able to treat her for the swollen legs.

It goes without saying that bone problems and joint problems often go hand in hand. I have often seen that arthritic joints were initially caused by a bone infection. I have been involved in a number of research projects in this field, and I have found it encouraging to have my philosophy confirmed. Arthritic joints are often caused by mental stress, originating in the emotional system and then affecting the endocrine system, for example stress at work, relationship problems or jealousy. When the glandular system becomes involved and imbalanced the joints may become stiff, and this is often a reflection of the person's mental condition. The same applies to a fracture or a broken bone. Unless we can dissociate our thoughts from our fear or concern about a fracture, the bone will be difficult to mend. On the other hand, much can be achieved by adopting a positive attitude. One such case I clearly remember concerned the father of an assistant of mine. She told me that her father had broken his wrist while out hill walking. Because he was a chiropodist he found it hard to accept that he was unable to use his hand and was upset by the fact that the wrist was encased in plaster. After about ten days his frustration got the better of him and he removed the plaster himself. He decided that he was strong enough to use his hand and wrist again, and he applied himself once again to his chiropody work.

I have seen on numerous occasions that arthritic patients have improved thanks to a positive attitude and the belief that they could influence their condition for the better. I have seen patients whose mobility and flexibility was badly impaired because of rheumatic conditions, and yet they were determined to continue to fend for themselves, rather than give in. These people I greatly admire, and will always do my utmost to help them. Despite the pain, they still keep fighting. In the research projects in which I have taken part, I have sometimes been mystified: I have seen two people with identical medical problems, of which one will improve, while the condition of the other does not change. The improvement cannot always be explained by that person having a stronger immune system, but I suspect that it is more to do with their positive attitude and determination of spirit.

I have been astounded by some of the stories of the survivors of concentration camps after the Second World War. These people were no longer physically strong, but mentally some had a single-minded determination to stay alive despite their inhumane treatment and loathsome environment. Many who appeared to be physically strong enough to endure the hardships failed to survive, while those with the mental determination succeeded in doing so.

Determination in rheumatic people can be the answer to their recovery. Joints are very much affected by the influences from within and from without. It is sad to see the effects of arthritis, which can be found even among the younger generation. This is a condition that is inherent in many people. Some pathological changes, usually occurring after middle-age, become very much part of life. Animals experience such problems too, and it is even seen in fish. Arthrosis, a degenerative process affecting the cartilage, is not an uncommon condition. It happens in the joints and it is important to take immediate action when this becomes apparent. Nowadays, we are beginning to gain a clearer understanding of the causes of arthrosis, rheumatism and arthritis. Although there can be hereditary and environmental factors, there is no doubt that these conditions are primarily influenced by nutritional factors. I was greatly encouraged when I started to work with some new findings on amino acids, such as glucosamine sulphate. When used in the treatment of osteoarthritis its effect on the forming of new cartilage is astonishing. This aminomonosaccharide is found in the joint cartilage and consists of glucose, an amine (nitrogen and two molecules of hydrogen) and sulphur. Another cartilage component, chondroitin sulphate, is also used in the treatment of arthritic conditions. Glucosamine sulphate, already recognised as an effective treatment for arthritis, is also proving to be of great help for arthrosis, and I have been excited by the encouraging results I have seen in some of my patients who have taken part in studies. Under close supervision, I have prescribed the remedy ArMax together with Imperarthritica and Urticalcin to some of my patients, often with a very satisfactory outcome. An uncomplicated acid-free diet, introducing more alkaline foods, plus some of these remedies, has also provided great relief. The joints are affected by nutritional deficiencies. Golf and tennis elbows can be solved easily nowadays with manipulation or acupuncture treatment. But prevention is better than cure and underlying such conditions we often find that there is a zinc deficiency, just as in other cases there may be deficiencies of glucosamine sulphate. Once the deficiency has been diagnosed, we stand a much better chance of correcting the imbalance, and in doing so bring about a reduction in pain and discomfort.

One of my lecturers once said that medicine does not need to be complicated, if only we know the correct remedy for the complaint or disease. In the Book of Proverbs it is stated that 'anger is the rotting of bones'. A good humour and an optimistic and happy attitude can be of tremendous help to people. One should always be careful when treating joints. Heavy traction will only make things worse, whereas gentle traction is beneficial, as is trying to put the joint through its normal range of motion with the help of techniques such as ultrasound, sonic therapy, hydrotherapy, infra-red rays and hot packs. According to the medical textbooks on arthritis and associated rheumatic conditions, the basic answer is often found in metabolic disturbances caused by the inability of the body to make available or utilise the necessary biochemical elements from a balanced diet. Arthritis, also according to the textbooks, is caused by infections, allergies, or inherited problems. It is often found, for example, that there is infection in the cervix or the prostate. The many types of arthritic conditions may require different approaches, as their causes may vary. I have written two books on that subject alone, and even still, every day, I learn yet about more missing links. Science and the accumulation of knowledge never stands still. Dr Leonard Allan has certainly never stood still and I have always regarded him as one of my great mentors. We have covered a lot of ground together as will be apparent from his notes which are incorporated in this chapter.

The elimination of metabolic waste and the availability of the relevant nutritional elements are necessary for effective results from gentle manipulative therapy. Manipulative or soft-tisssue therapy provides a means of stimulating the movement of all body fluids, especially the lymph and cerebro-spinal fluids, thus giving the co-operative patient additional relief, even if not a complete cure. All too often the main problem is that patients do not give it sufficient time. They are too impatient.

Arthropic or rheumatoid arthritis shows up as an inflammatory manifestation in the joints. Joints affected by a stressful existence, or a situation where much time is spent on the feet – as in the case of the female patient described at the beginning of this chapter – develop a systemic condition, where joint infection is manifested by severe and uncomfortable swellings. Treatment of the affected joints can be no more than palliative while the infection is still active. As stated earlier, the infection can be in the cervix in women and in the prostate in men. If effective treatment is applied to either of these sources and the cause is successfully eradicated, this can halt the progress of the disease, whether the joints are treated or not. It is a well-known fact that inflammation of the cervix and prostatitis are forms of pelvic infection. When we trace rheumatic conditions to dysfunction of the ovaries, or in men to the gonads, we have proof that the endocrine system plays a part in these particular arthritic joint problems.

Degenerative, hypertrophic or osteoarthritic conditions are not usually associated with any form of bacterial toxaemia and cannot therefore be attributed to an infection. In some cases it is found that an endocrine imbalance plays some part in their aetiology. Whether the condition is due to a change of some sort or is a consequence of advancing age, it seems to remain incurable, although certain forms of treatment can alleviate the pain. The most common form is suffered by women and is known as menopausal arthritis, and this is amenable to certain forms of therapy.

It has been well documented that rheumatoid arthritis is much more common in women than it is in men. It usually occurs during the child-bearing period of life, between the ages of eighteen and forty-five. The most common history is that of ill health, either coinciding with, or preceding the onset of arthritis, perhaps dating back to childbirth or miscarriage, both of which may be the cause of infection in the cervix. It is also ascribed in some cases, especially in virgins, to acute specific fevers, and appendicitis is another factor that can cause an infection of the cervix. It has been established clinically that the patient is usually thin, often anaemic and that there might be a slight pyrexia or fever. The joint infection is polyarthritis when the main brunt is being borne by the smaller joints, such as the fingers, toes, wrists and ankles, although the larger joints may also be affected.

It is sad that since Dr Allan first wrote his notes, probably no more than fifteen years ago, the prevalence of juvenile arthritis and polyarthritis has increased beyond belief. The arthritis is often symmetrical. The finger ends are cold and atrophic and the patient often exhibits a peculiar dampness and clamminess of the hands and fingers. The affected joints are swollen and the fingers usually show a fusiform enlargement: this is a char-acteristic of infective arthritis, whilst nodular enlargements are indicative of osteoarthritis. Joints are usually stiff and movement is painful. In time, the resultant damage to the joints can produce permanent fixation, sometimes of the articular ends due to the pull of the tendons, and consequent hyper-immobility. Deformity is often the result and other deviations in the fingers and bony ankylosis is common. There is usually abdominal tenderness and the condition of the cervix varies according to the stage of the arthritis. It is very common to find an active infection with a discharge associated with tenderness in the fornix at the top of the vagina. Often, in long-standing cases, the cervix shows only the signs of past infections. It may show deformity and scars radiating from the source of old infections. With severe arthritis, often the only changes visible in an X-ray are raised fractions of bone ends, though there may be some diminution of joints. In cases of infective arthritis, the large joints, i.e. the hips, knees and vertebral column, usually display signs of inflammation in the new bone in the tendons attached to the joints. This inflammatory new bone is seen as a spur which is usually more dense than the normal bone. The true osteophytic growth, characteristic of osteoarthritis, is usually not as dense, but often shows the laminated structure of the true bone. We often see these particular problems just starting when minor infections go untreated.

There are five distinct modes of onset in women:

1. The joints are usually affected in two ways. Some show up on the X-ray as having been destroyed, while others show atrophy of the bones with dislocation, an indication that the fixed joints were affected early and that fixation occurred rapidly. Subsequently, the other joints became involved slowly and insidiously.

2. Sometimes the joints are involved insidiously, the resultant pain and swelling leading, over the years, to crippling conditions. Care must be taken that ankylosis does not occur in such situations.

3. A rheumatic-fever type of onset, which resembles rheumatic fever with sweating, joint pain, inflammation.

4. In the above type the actual onset of arthritis is preceded by months or even years of backache, vaginal discharge or miscarriage, where typical rheumatoid arthritis can be the cause.

5. The latter is the type usually associated with the menopause and is often confused with osteoarthritis owing to the age of the patient. In some cases of infective arthritis, if left untreated, the patient will steadily deteriorate, while others have frequent remissions.

In all cases first look for a possible infection. Infections can be treated with some homoeopathic and herbal remedies such as Echinaforce, Imperathritica, mentioned earlier, ArMax, Urticalcin and Oil of Evening Primrose.

As mentioned earlier, arthritis in men is less common than it is in women. In men the onset usually takes place during puberty, which shows a major difference in the age of incidence. Both the cervix and the prostate are often prone to infection. While the cervix runs an extra risk during childbirth and in a miscarriage, in men the prostate often becomes enlarged, degenerated and prone to infection after middle age. Thus it is also more likely for men to contract arthritis after middle age. Examination of the abdomen usually reveals some tenderness in the lower region, usually on one side only. The tender area is hypersensitive to pin pricks, the sensitive area encircling the body like a half belt, corresponding to the lower dorsal and the upper lumbar segments of the spinal cord. Examination of the prostate may reveal nothing abnormal, but if the prostate is tender on one side, there will be a tender area on the abdominal wall on the same side. There may be general prostate tenderness and the gland may feel hard in one lobe, or nodular. The physical signs are variable. Microscopic examination of any secretion is not often helpful, unless an infection is found. In homoeopathy we may review this symptom in the light of a miasma, which is a left-over from former inflammations, viruses or infections. The source of the miasma may even go back to a previous generation, if there is an arthritic history in families which can be traced to some infectious disease. The onset of arthritis in men is often characterised by a rapid involvement and fixation of the joints, followed by the slow development of ankylosing arthritis, or a slow, insidious onset in all the affected joints, or a rheumatic fever-type onset as in women. It could also be a backache prostatitis syndrome, the type which in women is due to an inflammation of the cervix. These are quite common and most start with an infection. Patients suffer from fatigue and listlessness, together with low backache and abdominal pain. Indigestion and other digestive complaints can also be other symptoms. Apart from backache, the other outstanding symptom is nervousness, and these cases are usually labelled neurasthenia.

Prostatitis is frequently present in men, although often undiagnosed. Hence the reason I tend to advocate Prostabrit and/or Prostasan in combination as a treatment for middle-aged men who have stiffness in the joints, or possibly the beginning of arthritis. In young men, where the symptoms of juvenile arthritis are diagnosed, the condition is often due to an unknown case of prostatitis. We also see with younger girls that these symptoms stem from a problem in the ovaries. The treatment for young men with Prostabrit and Prostasan is a good starting point, while in young women I tend to work with stronger remedies such as Phytobiotic and Ovasan or *Ovarium D3*.

Looking at osteoarthritis, this is usually a form of menopausal syndrome and is amenable to treatment. Normally it is associated with menstrual irregularities and also hyper-thyroidism. However, if it affects the joints, usually the larger joints, or the weight-bearing joints, the condition is more difficult to contain. The joints appear enlarged, probably due to the thickening of periarticular structures. Patients usually complain that the knee locks, and then spontaneously recovers, and often that the joint gives way. The joint cavity is usually extended, with an enlarged synovial membrane. Some ridging of the articular margin can be felt at an early stage, and rubbing of the patella on the underlying cartilage, where there is a sensation of roughness. X-rays often reveal lipping of the bone at the articular margins. This usually is due to endocrine disturbance.

The beginning and end of adult life are marked by a rearrangement in the balance of power between the ductless glands. The total effect of these rearrangements towards the end of life makes up one aspect of what we sometimes call senility. But osteoarthritis is a very common manifestation. In old age there is a liability to this form of arthritis in both sexes. The joint infection in women displays itself in symptoms of the menopause, which in passing leaves the arthritis in an arrested condition. The amount of damage to the joints depends on the length of time that the menopause has lasted. Shortening the time reduces the damage and mobilisation of the essential treatment is important.

Osteoarthritis responds well to glucosamine sulphate, known as the product GS1000, together with Alchemilla Complex, and Osteo-Care. I have found that the combination of these three remedies have been of great help to many of my patients.

All the spondylitic conditions are similar to chronic arthritis, and infective spondylitis can also be caused by infection, or intestinal gastric infection or even ulcerations. Unless the lymphatics and the intercellular spaces are treated, spondylitis can take a firm hold. The degenerative form of spondylitis, or spondylitis deformans, usually involves a change in the vertebral column, where inflammatory changes or calcifications can occur. Such conditions result in considerable pain and severe limitation of movement in the spine – the end result being a poker-back spine, nearly always associated with inflammatory changes in the sacro-iliac joints, which are often affected before the upper spine. This condition is even more commonly caused by infection. It is said that osteoarthritis of the spine is incurable, but draining the lymphatics seems to be a key to the success of any further treatment. Most spondylitic conditions can be treated with electro-acupuncture if the correct pressure points are brought into play. If the practitioner is well qualified and knows exactly at which points the patient's energy passes through, and in which direction, great improvement can be obtained. Following an acid-free diet or an elimination diet, together with a course of electro-acupuncture treatment, or moxabustion acupuncture, has proved beneficial in many cases.

By now the reader has probably understood why I have placed so much emphasis on the endocrine glands earlier in the book. That small gland, the pituitary gland, which is only marginally bigger than a pinhead, releases a hormone at the first sign of stress, sounding an alarm to the body. This hormone travels through the body, by way of the blood-stream, to two other small glands that lie between the kidneys at the back, called the adrenals. The adrenals pick up the hormone, triggering the release of further hormones, the chief of which is called cortisol, which we also know as cortisone. Messages are relayed to the nervous system to release the hormone adrenaline. The presence of these adrenal hormones in the blood informs the entire body that it is under threat. Thus by concentrating on the endocrine system, a practitioner can restore balance in this particular situation.

There is one vertebra I have not yet mentioned and this I have left on purpose. The bottom of the spine ends in the coccyx, which comprises three very small crystals that can be easily damaged in a fall. Whenever damage to the coccyx occurs, the entire spine is affected and a message is sent, reaching even the atlas, at the top end of the spine. When the coccyx is affected, this in turn affects the atlas. With many arthritic patients, not only might there be a problem in the glands, but often the coccyx is involved. This factor is sometimes ignored in its relation to the cause of disease, but there could be trouble if there is an articulation of the hinge joints, i.e. those that are capable of anterior and posterior movement. The muscles that are attached to the coccyx are the coccygeus, the levator ani, and the sphincter ani which move the coccyx anteriorly, while the gluteus maximus draws it posteriorly and laterally. The coccygeal nerve emerges between the first and second coccygeal segments. The filium terminale of the spinal cord is attached to the posterial surface of the coccygeal segments. Anterior to the coccyx is the ganglion of impar, which constitutes the inferior end of the ganglionic chain of the automatic nervous system. We often find that when the coccyx is in trouble it exerts pressure on the ganglion of impar. This, in turn, will result in disturbances of the involuntary function, which express themselves through diverse symptoms. Anterior displacement also places traction on the filium terminale, which in turn pulls on the entire spinal cord and may cause almost any symptoms of nervous origin. If the practitioner is capable and decides on palpation of the coccyx, it must be borne in mind that the tip of the sacrum may appear to be a displaced coccyx. In this event the sacrum should be corrected, which will at the same time correct the coccyx. In some cases the coccyx should be gently lifted to alleviate the pressure on the ganglion of impar. A good practitioner can do this successfully.

There are of course many joint conditions, many kinds of arthritic problems, of which I have only mentioned a few. Some are frequently overlooked, like some of the causes of arthritis in men and women. It is never possible to use a standard medicine to treat such problems, because the causes and symptoms are often dependent on the individual, but it should always be remembered that all joints, bones and muscles should work in harmony as one unit.

15

Healthy Muscles

Dr Andrew Still, the father of osteopathy, stated that his philosophy of manipulation is based on an absolute knowledge of each and every bone in the body, their several parts in articulation and their normal movements. He fully realised that motion to restore is the one outstanding force, that maintains itself normally, in all moveable parts, particularly the fascia and the tissue, and that this motion is the result of muscle contraction.

Our muscles account for 15 per cent of our total body weight. Striated muscles are organs of proto-plasmic cells, which are elongated to form fibres attached by both ends. Each muscle is covered by a membrane fascia. A stimulus to the cell in the central nervous system, or to its motor neurone, originates an impulse resulting in tonal waves and contractions. Muscles possess excitability, i.e. they contract when stimulated directly, mechanically or otherwise. They require a stimulus to contract and a stimulus to relax. Motion is the first and only evidence of life and is the most widespread of all vital activities. There is no life without movement. Where there is diminished movement, there is disease; where there is no movement, there is death. All movement of the body, skeletal and visceral, as well as of the blood and tissue fluids, is affected through muscle contraction. A resting muscle contracts between five and fifty times per second. Active muscles may reach three thousand contractions per second tonal waves. Contraction of the heart muscle pumps the blood from the heart to the cells. The skeletal muscles return the veinous blood to the heart, and muscle contraction is necessary for its own blood circulation.

As I have said before, muscles move bones. Bones will not move without muscles. The human frame is expertly formed, each muscle having its own inbuilt tension, its own inbuilt ability to contract or relax its fibres. Every part of the body is dependent on muscle and life's processes could not continue to function without muscles. Their physical condition is a good indication of the state of the muscles. Vitality is indicative of good muscle tone and the opposite is also true, when muscles lose their tone and become flabby. You should have sufficient interest in your health to make a detailed study of body muscles, as it will repay you a thousandfold. Study the controls through the nerve fibres, as these affect their contraction and relaxation. Whatever the name given to diseases, and there are more than a thousand such names, muscles are the basis of these aches and pains. A contracted muscle is a working muscle. It uses up nervous energy, consumes sugar and produces lactic acid — and this is the ultimate cause of fatigue. To produce a state of relaxation in muscle tissue, apply pressure with the thumbs at both the origin and insertion of the muscle. This serves to drain the accumulated acids from the muscle and allows fresh nourishment to enter the fibres. The pressure should not be maintained for more than about ten to twenty seconds. In this way, normal muscle tone will soon be established, probably due to a vibration of the muscle itself produced by the discontinuance of the excitation. The cellular and intercellular tensions must be corrected so as to remove all strain and thus restore the muscle to its maximum efficiency by eliminating fatigue.

Contraction of the muscles is caused by nerve impulses passing, via a spinal trunk nerve, to the nerve endings of the muscle. In a normal healthy person this contraction, followed by relaxation mainly due to exercise, gives what is known as muscle tone. Such voluntary exercise improves the metabolism and increases the circulation of the blood which flows through the muscle, and thus the muscle is permanently strengthened. When the nerves, through disease or injury, are no longer able to conduct these nerve impulses, in the majority of cases muscle contraction is impossible. When a muscle remains contracted, the result is fatigue, pain and other harmful effects. Its supply of oxygen is cut off, affecting blood and lymph that are squeezed out of the tissues.

People talk glibly about tension. What they have in mind is muscular tension. A muscle is capable of contraction and relaxation, but a muscular spasm is a different matter. The blood is squeezed out of a spastic muscle, so that oxygen cannot get to the tissues. Nature gives us a warning through what we know as pain.

Everything in nature is in a state of molecular tension; otherwise man, the moon, planets and other visible objects would disintegrate and fly off into space. Everything is in motion. Nothing stands still. Stillness is death, destruction and change.

Tension, therefore, is a natural function and state of being. It is the most important factor in physical life. It is responsible for the birth of a form, controlling the harmonious distribution of energy through its body.

It is the 'state of tension' that preserves the integrity of a form. The molecular construction of anything, be it animate or inanimate, is dependent upon this natural law of tension. Whether you call it Life, Health or Cosmic Energy, it is the factor that keeps molecules from flying off into space. The tensile strength of a human cell is an electrical phenomenon and is allied to its frequency or rate of vibration. When this is altered by faulty diet or even microbic invasion, the frequency and tension is altered, resulting in disease or disharmony. Tension, as we know it, is muscular in nature, whether it be produced by the cold weather (when we automatically tense our muscles), emotional stimuli, etc. We all know what happens when a muscle remains in a state of tension for any length of time, so I will not go into this.

Going back to tension, inner conflict and emotional upsets: these factors, when persistent, actually precipitate soluble calcium from the bloodstream into the joints and bursae, the result being arthritis, rheumatism, lumbago and other health problems. Therefore I repeat that tension ends in visceral motor tension and deposits. Mind has become matter. This is a negative miracle. The positive miracle is to supplant the latter with joy, happiness and the ideal conditions for survival.

Therapy has as its basis the observation that pressure on a cellulome, also called a trigger point, has a healing effect. Apart from its local or remote anaesthetic action, a cellulome, which is the focal point of an irritation somewhere, usually on the surface of the body, can cause many different diseases and pain syndromes. Sustained pressure on these alarm points can check inflammation and it is also claimed that this can cure the disease itself. Sustained pressure on a cellulome characterised by a hyper-aesthetic spot or zone on the skin will influence the organs lying deeper within the body. There are a number of muscle triggers, or points that have an area-preferred pain. If we analyse these pains and apply gentle pressure to these muscle triggers, the pains can be eliminated or at least relieved. Always remember that within every man or woman there is a force which directs and controls the entire course of life. It can heal every infection and ailment to which mankind is susceptible. Remember too that most diseases have one common origin, and this origin is none other than a toxic condition which can result from food fermentation, and that from the first attack to the time of the cure of the patient, this original cause has a greater influence upon the condition of the patient than the symptoms that are so frequently treated. Continuing emphasis is given to the importance of the blood supply to the brain, especially the emotional areas, due primarily to the excessive sympathetic stimulation of the vascular system supplying the emotional centres of the brain. This excessive stimulation causes the musculature to contract, a state which, if prolonged, invariably results in disease. The daily bombardment of negative stimuli, which accompanies us all from the cradle and persists throughout our life, will also accompany us to the grave. Man possesses an electric field complete with its own sub-power stations and a convenient collection of power points and fuses spread over the entire surface of the body. Visceral and body tension produces short circuits, known as trigger points. Manipulation and acupuncture restore the broken fuse, thereby allowing a spontaneous cure to follow.

I have often been amazed to see how practitioners with a sound knowledge of the muscular system, by using the correct trigger points, can free patients from spasms, enabling a fresh blood supply to permeate the stagnant tissue. Strong muscles are necessary to move strong bones. With the sacro-iliac joint, for example, which is a mystery to even the best orthopaedic surgeon, we can see the extent to which the muscle is involved with this bone. In serious problems affecting the sacro-iliac joint, if we work on certain trigger points towards the joint in the muscle, the patient can be accorded much relief. Muscle balance is of the highest importance, because as long as the muscle remains in a state of tension, spasms cannot be relieved.

Every time I pass the hallway to my office I see a framed saddle-cloth which once belonged to one of the most famous horses in Britain. The horse and his rider were both brought to me after some trials, where the horse had been injured during a fall. The rider had also injured herself as she had come off the saddle during the fall only to be pinned to the ground underneath the horse. The veterinary surgeon had told the rider that it would be many months before the horse would be fit again. She was very upset by this and had explained that the horse was supposed to take part in the European Championships in Germany. A friend of hers who had also attended the trials recommended that she should seek my advice. Thus they arrived at my clinic and waited until I had finished with my patients. I noticed immediately that both the horse and the rider were suffering from severe muscular spasms. I shall never forget the gratitude in the big soft eyes of the horse when I managed to relieve these spasms that were racking his body. Then I treated the rider. There was a similarity between their injuries. I used acupuncture on certain trigger points and gave both the rider and the horse some homoeopathic remedies: Arnica for healing and Symphosan for external application. After four treatment sessions both horse and rider were once again showing some of their old stamina. They were able to compete in the European Championships in Germany and won. I was given the saddle-cloth as a souvenir and token of gratitude for contributing to that occasion.

Any muscular problem should be given proper attention. Muscles are important because they give motion to life, or if they cease, stillness to death. Muscles are strengthened by exercise and by feeding them with the necessary nutrients. As well as the manipulative treatment and the natural remedies for both horse and rider, I also prescribed a high supplementary dose of vitamin B complex. This is because the B group of vitamins is a collection of essential nutrients that have certain characteristics in common. They are all non-protein, nitrogen-containing, water-soluble substances found in food sources such as brewer's yeast, meat, whole grains, cereals and vegetables. While they are chemically distinct from one another, the ways in which the B vitamins work in the body are closely interrelated. For example: the metabolisms of folic acid and vitamin B_{12} are closely connected; vitamin B_2 is required for the activation of vitamin B_6; and vitamin B_3 can be manufactured from other dietary agents provided there is adequate vitamin B_6. The vitamin B complex functions in the body as a *group* of vitamins. It is essential for the release of energy from food and for the metabolism of fats and protein. The group contributes to the maintenance of healthy skin, hair, eyes, mouth and liver and the production of haemoglobin. The correct functioning of the brain and nervous system requires that vitamin B complex vitamins are regularly available from the diet.

We must not forget folic acid, which is essential for a healthy muscular system. Folic acid helps in the formation of iron-carrying haemoglobin needed by red blood cells. It is also needed for the metabolism of DNA and RNA – the nucleic acids that are at the source of cell life. It is also involved with the production of digestive acid, with a healthy appetite and with periods of extra bio-activity, such as during pregnancy and growth. By feeding the muscular system with the correct nutrients we can strengthen the bones and joints and support the overall skeletal system.

A good balance should be found, however, because overdoing it is not helpful either, and occasionally I have to correct the excessive intake of such supplements, especially by people involved in weight-lifting.

Exercise is just as important for the muscular system as the correct nutrition. It should always be remembered that if people force their muscles in unaccustomed exercise, it may result in the need for a visit to an osteopath or chiropractitioner. I have seen too many patients with serious muscular problems caused by suddenly deciding, after years of following a sedentary lifestyle, that they should take up physical exercise. Exercise is all very well, but common sense can sometimes be thrown out of the window, and instead of slowly building up a fitness programme, these people throw themselves in at the deep end. Here again the three bodies of man come into play. It is not certain to what extent muscular problems can be attributed to nutritional inadequacy or a deficiency of specific ingredients in the diet. With serious problems such as muscular dystrophy, which is characterised by progressive wasting of the muscle fibres, there are still some big question marks. However, I have some patients who are not in a progressive state, and who take care of themselves, and they still attend my clinic, even after twenty years. A positive spirit has been able to help them through.

Amino acids are widely recommended in some cases of muscular waste. Amino acids are the building blocks from which the giant protein molecules are composed through the condensation reaction between amino and carboxyl groups. Each amino acid contains nitrogen as well as carbon, hydrogen and oxygen and they form a large class of organic compounds. Isomeric forms of the amino acids can exist, as mirror-images of one another. Since it is protein that provides the structure for all living things, the importance of amino acids cannot be over-emphasised. Amino acids may be linked together in an almost indefinite variety of sequences to form more than 50,000 proteins, of which 20,000 are enzymes. They contain about 16 per cent nitrogen and it is this that distinguishes them from carbohydrates and fats.

Amino acids such as threonine or L-methionine have proved very beneficial in the treatment of muscle disorders. Carnitine is another invaluable amino acid and a constituent of the muscles and liver. It can be synthesised from lysine in the presence of vitamin C, and its most important known metabolic function is to transport long chains of fatty acids into the mitochondria of the muscle cells for oxidation. Carnitine is essential for optimal growth and development. Cardiac muscle is especially dependent upon this mechanism as an important source of metabolic energy. Additionally, carnitine plays a role in the production of heat (thermogenesis) in the brown adipose tissue and in the regulation of glucogenesis (glucose production).

The essential amino acid phenylalanine exists as two enantiomers 'd' and 'l', both of which play a role in the response of the body and mind to physical and chemical challenges. The 'dl' form is best utilised by the body. Phenylalanine is known to safeguard the body's natural production of endorphins and encephalins, which are soothing substances released by

145

the brain. The metabolism of phenylalanine requires vitamin B_6 (pyridoxine), vitamin C, niacin (or vitamin B_3), iron and copper, hence the composition of a remedy called DLPA Complex.

Yet another remedy in which I have great faith is called Protein Deficiency Formula. The contribution made by proteins to the energy value of most well-balanced diets is usually between 10 and 15 per cent of the total and seldom exceeds 20 per cent. Whereas the fat in the body can be derived from dietary carbohydrates and the carbohydrates from proteins, the proteins of the body are inevitably dependent for their formation and maintenance on the amino acid supply in food or food supplements. Proteins are constantly used by the body for its normal function, growth and repair. Many factors influence the efficiency of the digestive system in breaking down proteins into amino acids for absorption. Factors such as illness, stress, old age and the reduced ability to secrete digestive enzymes may result in poor digestion of protein. By supplementing the diet with amino acids, the body can be saved the necessary step of digesting (or breaking down) dietary protein to obtain them.

These supplements have contributed to the return to health of several of my patients. It begs the question of whether there is a missing link regarding the wider availability of amino acids in their natural form in certain countries, for in those countries diseases such as multiple sclerosis or muscular dystrophy are very rare. It never ceases to amaze me that, despite our advanced scientific knowledge, there is so much that we still do not know. It is essential that the secrets of nature are scientifically investigated, because I am sure that there is an awful lot more to learn.

In front of me I have a copy of a newspaper article about a typical example of a man who was under great emotional pressure. When he came to my clinic he told me that four years previously he had been told that he was suffering from the fatal and incurable disease called MND (motor neurone disease). There was certainly a stiffness in his muscles and also clear signs of muscle waste. After I had performed some tests I began to doubt the previous diagnosis. One could not help but feel sorry for him, because his relationship with his wife was suffering under the strain, although she was determined to stand by him. He saw how other MND sufferers were slowly deteriorating, becoming wheelchair-bound, and preparing themselves for their demise. An article in his local paper was devoted to the mental and emotional devastation of this patient and others like him. Then, in his own words, like a miracle, the death sentence hanging over him was lifted. He received a letter from the hospital chiefs apologising for the distress and anxiety caused to him, when after more tests it was concluded that he was *not* suffering from MND. Although he is clearly not well, and is suffering from an illness which I believe to be neurological, he has made progress. Muscle waste is indeed a very serious situation. Our muscles are very important to us and when we complain that our muscles feel tired or tense, we should consider whether we are physically or emotionally tired, as our muscles are the first indication of the reason. We have all experienced a little flutter in the eye, when the eye muscles become fatigued, often after a tiring or emotionally draining time. Even these little spasms of the eye muscles convey a warning that it is time for rest or relaxation. Harmony should be regained in order to allow the muscles to function correctly so that the bones and joints can be kept moving, and keep us fit and healthy.

I remember a female patient who worked in the civil service. She was experiencing a lot of stress at work and emotional tension at home and developed the condition of polymyelgia rheumatica. This is not an easy condition to treat and yet she is a very happy and relaxed person today. I told her that she had to learn to relax, and enter into harmony with her work and her relationship at home. In order to help her I gave her some remedies and advised her to change her diet. She was in need of help because her nervous system was very overworked. Unfortunately, polymyelgic rheumatica is a growing problem, and I am sure this is because of the stress factor involved. This lady conscientiously followed my advice and changed her diet. I gave her electro-acupuncture treatment, and she took Oil of Evening Primrose, Imperarthritica and Symphosan, and later I also prescribed ArMax and garlic capsules. Her progress was slow, but I alternated the electro-acupuncture with moxabustion treatment, for which I also used a homoeopathic remedy in the needle, and after every treatment session she felt better. She had told me that her position at work was very demanding and that she had been barely able to cope when this condition brought her down. Now that she is no longer plagued by the back and shoulder pain that accompany this condition, she looks forward to going to work. She feels that she is more than capable of doing her job to her satisfaction. This again shows that by achieving harmony, and maintaining the right perspective, with a positive outlook and determination, people can overcome their condition.

16

Healthy Eyes

You may remember that I have already pointed out that there are seven endocrine glands, seven basic steps in the muscial octave and seven colours in the solar spectrum. There also are seven layers of light receptors in the eye retina. The relatively new diagnostic method known as iris diagnosis, or iridology, has opened up new horizons in alternative medicine. Through this technique, practitioners are able to use the body's most accurate natural X-ray system – the eye – to determine how the life force moves and operates within the body. Every abnormality in the physical body and every perversity in the mental body is clearly impressed upon the iris, and through its records we stand exposed to each other as though we were living in a glasshouse into which he who looks and knows may see.

On 26 January 1826, near Budapest in Hungary, a great discovery was made by an eleven-year-old child called Ignatz Peczely. While playing in the garden, the young boy captured an owl and in the struggle that ensued the bird sustained a broken leg. After the owl had been subdued, the observant boy noticed a white cloud in the lower part of the bird's iris, on the same side as the injured leg. When the leg had healed, he noticed that a black speck circumscribed by white lines had replaced the former cloud. He recalled the incident later, when as a physician he was called upon to treat a fracture in a man's leg. He proceeded at once to examine the man's iris and immediately noticed a curious cloud in the patient's eye, similar to the one he had observed in the bird's eye. From that time he continued his investigations, which led to his discovery of specific areas of the iris, that correspond to organs in the body. This led to the foundation of this valuable diagnostic method, iridology.

To those who are familiar with the science of iris diagnosis, the sympathetic wreath is so-called on account of its shape. It represents the area of the sympathetic nervous system in the iris. It is seen near and around the pupil, as a white circle in the iris, though it may in some cases be overshadowed by the encumbrance of a drug discolouration. For any deviation in the normal regularity of the circle we usually find a corresponding irregularity in the function of the organ towards which it points. Thus, by careful analysis of irregularities in the sympathetic wreath it is possible to detect points of great diagnostic value which may otherwise remain hidden. A well-trained iridologist can see at a glance which organ is affected, and more important still, after each touch of the probe or stylet, what progress has been made.

On careful examination, a greenish/blue colour in the eye reveals the seven layers of light receptors in the retina of the eye. In fact, we can see the seven divisions on the physical plane, which has seven colours, like a rainbow. The form of energy we know as sound has seven notes in music and the same note recurs in each key, only it is of a higher or lower pitch according to which side of the scale is selected. A well-known scientist, Dr Dinshah P. Ghadiali, has made a great contribution to medicine with his studies of the science of colours and light. He found, after years of research, that red, yellow and blue are not the fundamental colours of life. He established the true triad of primary colours of light, i.e. red, green, violet, and the triad of secondary colours, i.e. yellow, blue and magenta. He formulated his method of treatment on twelve colours of vibrant light: red, orange, yellow, lemon, green, turquoise, blue, indigo, violet and a hidden portion of the rainbow, such as purple, magenta and scarlet. It seems that magenta is the most significant colour frequency in the evolution. In his writings Dr Ghadiali mentions that just as the musical scale has seven main tones and five semi-tones, making a total of twelve – for example on the piano keyboard, seven white keys and five black keys – so can the spectrum of light be analysed into the seven main colours and five semi-tone colours. These again make a total of twelve and each colour vibrates and oscillates at its own distinctive speed of wreath formation. Colour is a most valued gift of nature and it does not bear thinking about what life would be like if we could only see things in black and white. Yet scientists have failed to analyse the recent advances in our understanding of colour. Even in ancient times colour was greatly appreciated, valued and understood, and in many parts of the world, particularly in Greece and Egypt, historical traces remain of temples of light and colour.

It was not my intention in this book to write specifically about light and colour, but I do want to make sure it is understood that every endocrine gland in the body reacts to a specific colour, and how the retina will reveal, through its seven layers of light, what is happening elsewhere in the body. This is the key to the importance of the eye as a diagnostic tool to a physician, as it gives him the means to look inside the body. Here again, the drive towards mental, physical and emotional harmony is of fundamental importance. Not only do the eyes express what is going on inside the body, but they can also reflect what is perceived outside. With the eyes we can express our feelings, which are sometimes more difficult to express in words. Sometimes, too, the feelings expressed through the eyes might belie the spoken word. Furthermore, we have all heard the saying 'Beauty is in the eye of the beholder'. Love is blind, and this means that even though we may recognise faults in a person we love, this does not affect the emotional bond of love.

I have watched people with myopic sight concentrate on a particular aspect of their surroundings, instead of giving the impression of taking in a larger picture. This became obvious during a test that was done with the co-operation of thirty people. They had been placed in a dark room and when the lights were switched on they were asked to say what they saw first. Almost every person had a different answer. This shows that we frequently see what we want or expect to see. I am explaining this because I want to make sure that the three bodies of man, which are part of all our lives, are seen subjectively.

Bearing in mind the three bodies of man, people with impaired vision or other sight problems are often advised to try some visualisation techniques. This is because the optic nerve, when it leaves the eyeball, travels to the centres of visualisation and imagination, and to the cross-section of the medulla. The nerves branch out from this point, making their way to the spinal column. One pair connects to the third cervical vertebra, or between the third and fourth cervicals, at about the middle part of the neck. From the third cervical, the current will continue down to the heart and stomach. We should consider three things: first, we must consider the condition of our soul; then we must consider the condition of our stomach, and then our circulation.

If you place your thumb and forefinger on the bridge of the nose and forehead, you will soon notice that any tension leaves the eyes. Next, place the fingers on the back of the neck, on the bone lying midway between the shoulders and skull. If you find a sore spot, you will know that the bone is out of position or under stress. This stressed or misaligned bone is one possible cause of poor sight and a number of other eye problems. With continuous treatment you may notice that the cervical vertebra moves back into place without any physical assistance. Many people have managed to rebuild their sight with the help of these simple movements.

Calcium phosphate re-establishes the expression of the tissue that extends from the bridge of the nose, and between the eyes, back into the brain connecting with the optic nerve and with the centres of imagination and visualisation. Through the functioning of these tissues we can project any object – real or imagined. To visualise is to see. A man imagines that he has some unwanted condition in his body or brain, and through the centre of his imagination he builds it up until it manifests itself in reality. Or, vice versa, he can use the same power to create a good or sound part of the brain or body from illness. He can manifest a toothache into a cancer. By the same power, the problems can be removed, if the desire and belief is strong enough.

Visualisation techniques can be highly effective. Remember the saying about the three monkeys: hear no evil, see no evil and speak no evil. Positive thoughts are very important. Visualise that your problems can be overcome.

My mother's family had a tendency towards very poor eyesight and from childhood I have struggled with a form of colour blindness. I have learned to understand how important colours are for the eye, and the last thing I could have accepted was a colourless world. Instead of accepting that fact I have mentally strived to overcome it and therefore I know as well as anyone the value of good eyesight.

I am called upon to treat an increasing number of patients with conjunctivitis. This condition often occurs in people who are experiencing emotional problems or conflicts, and is not always caused by infection. For this reason, whenever I see patients with conjunctivitis I will take time to discover whether their condition is indeed caused by an infection, or if that person is subject to stress. A characteristic of this condition is red and bloodshot eyes, and the nervous habit of rubbing the eyes needs to be controlled so as not to exacerbate this. *Euphrasia*, or eyebright, is a herb with a soothing effect, and I often recommend that patients take five drops of the remedy Euphrasiasan three times a day. How wonderful are the healing gifts of nature; there even exist herbs and plants with properties that will heal and strengthen organs such as the liver and kidneys. These organs belong to the emotional body and dysfunction of these organs often results in blurred or impaired vision. Bathing the eyes with diluted Euphrasiasan is often very refreshing, and a similar effect can be obtained using some chamomile water or Occulosan eye drops.

For general strengthening of the eyes, in all conditions, I often advise patients to use the remedy Vision Essentials, because it contains bilberry extract, which I have always found to be very helpful. This remedy also contains the correct amount of vitamin A. We should be aware that, while vitamins can be of great help, they must be used in the right proportions, because overdosing with vitamins can cause an allergic reaction. Most people know that vitamin A is very beneficial for our eyesight, but it should be remembered that too much of this vitamin can actually be detrimental. Often it is advised to eat plenty of carrots, and this is indeed good advice because carrots are rich in vitamin A; however, I know of a man who drank twelve bottles of carrot juice a day, and this caused irreversible liver damage. We should always use our common sense.

Outwardly the body gives all the signs and symptoms of disease, and we must make sure that these signals are correctly interpreted. A little while ago a patient in her teens told me that she had blurred vision. She told me that sometimes her vision was totally blurred, but that it was not constant. I asked her if she was often thirsty, and when I took a sample to check her blood sugar level, it gave me a reading of over 18. As the normal reading should be in the region of 4 to 8, it immediately became clear that she had an inordinately high blood sugar level and should be treated for diabetes. Indeed, her eyes had suffered and I prescribed some supplementary vitamin C, as this is required for the synthesis of collagen and other connective tissue in the eyes. Bilberry extract was also helpful, together with a remedy based on the periwinkle plant. As an interesting aside, I have heard that in the Second World War, British Air Force pilots and navigators consumed large quantities of bilberries, because it was known to be helpful for their eyes.

I have also found that supplementary vitamin C can help in the treatment of glaucoma. This condition also seems to be more common nowadays, and when it is accompanied by pain I not only prescribe vitamin C, but also recommend Arterioforce (fifteen drops, three times a day) and acupuncture treatment. Glaucoma can be a serious problem and therefore a doctor or specialist must be consulted, not only to find relief for the pain, but because if it remains untreated, it can seriously endanger the eye-sight. This condition is caused by pressure on the eyeball as a result of excess fluid. The tension and worries of our life may contribute to the development of such a condition: physical and mental strain, caused by working in artificial light, using visual display units and watching television, are all factors that increase stress on the eyes. Just as with many other conditions, the glaucoma patient should make sure that he or she takes plenty of exercise in the fresh air, to counter the detrimental effects of these artificial influences. I have already pointed out that the pineal gland — the conductor of the endocrine system, and our aerial to the cosmos — is closely connected to the eyes. Transmitted messages received by the pineal gland will influence the condition of the eyes. Fortunately, surgery is not always the only answer in the treatment of a glaucoma, because some of the above-mentioned remedies can be of great help. I must re-emphasise, however, that the advice of a medical practitioner should always be sought. The minerals zinc and selenium have a positive role to play in the treatment of such conditions. I have seen some dramatic improvements that can be attributed to their use even in cases where patients showed a slight detachment of the eye retina, or more general degeneration.

Zinc is an essential trace mineral, and the principal role of any trace element is that of promoting the catalytic action of enzymes. Zinc is an invaluable mineral, which plays a role in dehydrogenation and peptidase processes. Zinc is also an integral component of insulin – the hormone used for the treatment of diabetes – and is essential for all protein synthesis in the body. Any extra physical or mental demands made on the body can increase the need for zinc or cause our bodies to lose zinc, where phytate and fibre-rich foods inhibit the absorption of zinc from food.

Selenium is also an essential trace mineral and a supplier of antioxidant nutrients. Along with vitamins C and E, which are antioxidants in their own right, selenium contributes to the raw materials from which the body makes glutathione peroxidase as well as another enzyme that converts thyroxines into the more active tri-iodothyroxine.

A cataract develops when the crystalline lens or its capsule becomes opaque, causing partial or total blindness. There are herbal lotions available for treating this condition, and fortunately science has become very advanced in this area. I remember that when I was still very young, my grandmother had an operation to remove a cataract, and this was in the very early days of such techniques. Nowadays, science has moved rapidly ahead and cataracts are treated by laser, with a tremendous success rate. However, surgery is not always necessary, but it is thought that if a cataract interferes with vision, it should be removed. Often the cataract is no more than an indication that something should be done, and if this condition is treated in time, the need for surgery may be avoided.

Just as colours fade in the sunlight, so can ultraviolet light damage eyes, and it is worth remembering that it is not only bright sunlight that can cause strain or damage to the eyes, but so can interior lighting. To minimise the effects, take antioxidants such as vitamins C and E, zinc and/or selenium supplements, and an enzyme preparation such as Glutiathone, Euphrasiasan or Vision Essential. However, I remind the reader that in the case of eye strain or complaints you should always seek medical advice. People with eye conditions will already know that smoking has a detrimental effect. Any time spent in a smoky atmosphere will increase the discomfort.

I remember one patient, whom I came to like very much. We first met when he came to see me about a totally unrelated condition, but I soon discovered that he had lost the sight in one of his eyes, making him totally dependent on the sight in his remaining eye. Unfortunately, due to strain, the condition of that eye was deteriorating rapidly. In our clinic we have a strict no-smoking policy and I watched him getting out of the car one day, his pipe dangling out of the corner of his mouth, his eyes creased to avoid the spiralling smoke from irritating the eye in which there was still some vision. When he was in my consulting room and I asked him, he admitted that he was an inveterate pipe smoker, and rarely removed the pipe from his mouth. I explained the damage he was doing to his remaining eye with this smoke, and after having first changed the pipe to the other corner of his mouth, he eventually gave up smoking. He was a very happy man when he realised that with his own action and with the help of some natural remedies, his eyesight was improving.

Cataract sufferers are advised to take Hyperisan (twice daily, ten drops before meals), together with five tablets of Urticalcin and Aesculaforce (twice daily after meals). Their diet should include plenty of carrots, bilberries and fruit juices. They will also find that warm compresses on the eyes are soothing. This advice also applies for what is called 'green cataract', in which case it is also recommended to follow a rice diet and take fifteen drops of Nephrosolid twice a day in a cup of Golden Grass Tea. For a 'grey cataract' the above advice is also valid, but on alternate days a tablet of *Belladonna D4* and *Phosphorus D6* should be taken.

I also remember the case of a young man with a corneal ulcer. He was a very keen clay pigeon shot, and his eye condition placed him under a lot of strain. We started the treatment with supplementary vitamins, minerals and trace elements, and I included Petasan, which is an excellent remedy for ulcers in general. Finally, he was advised to use Occulosan drops and Euphrasiasan. He was so grateful when it became clear how much his condition had improved and it was fascinating to watch the white patch of the ulcer gradually turning dark again.

An eye infection can have much wider repercussions than its effect on the eye itself. It usually affects the whole system. If such an inflammation occurs occasionally, remember that fasting, or an all-fruit diet can be beneficial, as can hot fermentations applied behind the ears, and chamomile compresses over the eyes. This advice applies for any inflammatory eye condition such as iritis, keratitis and retinitis. Some of the exercises outlined at the end of this chapter are also very helpful for these conditions.

A stye indicates a toxic condition in the system, and apart from applying fermentations, bathing the eye with Epsom salts can help and sometimes dabbing the affected area with diluted Molkosan, as well as taking Nephrosolid and Golden Grass Tea internally. A further homoeopathic remedy called *Podophyllum D3* is also recommended for styes.

Inflammation of the optic nerve is a further condition which greatly worries me, because I have had to treat so many multiple sclerosis patients with complaints caused by such an inflammation. I need not tell you that the eye is the most sensitive and vulnerable part of the anatomy. Inflammation of the optic nerve can lead to very serious problems indeed and should be treated immediately. If medical advice is not sought it is asking for bigger problems, and I have seen many MS patients where I suspect that their problems would have been much less severe if they had come to see me sooner, or if they had consulted an eye specialist right away.

Remember that visual complaints such as double or blurred vision are an alarm signal that something is not right. If proper advice is received early enough we can protect ourselves from serious disease. The other day I met a scientist who was under treatment for his eyesight problems from a highly regarded specialist in this field. The patient's condition started to deteriorate and he was very cynical about alternative treatment, but I reassured him that I would not keep him as a patient for longer than necessary, and if I felt that I could not help him I would let him know. I gave him acupuncture and laser treatment and some of the remedies mentioned earlier. His sight improved and eventually his specialist told him that the pressure behind the eyes was now completely normal, but he could not explain why. I was happy to get this feedback, because I knew that he did not feel positive about alternative treatment, but when he noticed his initial gradual improvement, he seemed to change his mental outlook and become less sceptical, and so the treatment became more effective.

One of my very best friends, who lives in India, was very concerned that his wife might be losing her sight. He travelled all over the world in search of a cure for her, and finally he came to spend some time with my family. I took her to the best eye specialist I knew of, but unfortunately we learned it was too late. At one point they thought that she had regained some vision, but this proved to be only temporary. It is with this case in mind that I stress again that such conditions must not be left untreated. To keep the vision clear, our physical, mental and emotional balance is of the greatest importance.

My friend Leonard Allan has worked out a self-help programme for various eye conditions, which I have found to be of great help and, with his permission, I will close this chapter with a summary of his instructions:

Eye discomfort, eye strain, burning sensations and other dysfunctions can be greatly relieved by any of the following methods:

1. Rub a little mentholatum on the eyelid, then apply a hot wet compress – reheat it several times. Apply also to the back of the neck, high under the occipital ridge. Once in a while, cold packs will be of great benefit. This is a simple way of breaking up strain.

2. Palming: Close your eyes – shutting out all the light. Cross your hands – lay the back of one hand into the palm of the other – rest them on your nose – place the heel of the hand on the cheek bone. No pressure on the eyes, this is an exercise of *rest*. The eye is the organ of light and is working every second it is open and exposed to light. Palming is conscious relaxation, or *rest*.

3. Bathe the eyes by submerging the face in a pan of cold water – open the eyes – roll them around – repeat several times. Or use an eye bath in the same way. A little salt, boric acid (powder or crystals) or Epsom salts in the water is soothing, cooling and good for mild irritations. The eye bath should be continued until the eyes feel comfortable.

4. Massage of the eyeball is beneficial in that it stirs up the blood and lymph streams, improving circulation. With the heel of the hand or tips of the fingers, light pressure is applied to the eyeball with a rotary movement, first one way and then the other. This is very stimulating to the eye tissues and is not harmful to the eye if done within reason. It is very good for tired eyes after a hard day's work – astigmatism – phorias – weak eyes – poor visual acuity, etc.

5. Exercises: Most eye trouble is functional in old or young and is due to maladjustment of the visual mechanism. Vision is a dual function – each eye must perform like the other. Very often the muscles controlling the movement of the eyes must be retrained to work in co-ordination with each other before visual training can be started.

6. Roll the eyes as far right as possible – then left – then up – then down – then in a circle to the right – reverse – then rest. Hold your head in a steady straightforward position, facing forward, throughout. Do not

turn the head – turn the eyes. Repeat this exercise six to eight times, two or three times a day. Take it easy. Do not overdo it.

7. Look at the end of your nose – then look away across the street at some distant object or look at the point of a pencil held in front of the eyes at different distances. Practise the change of focus intermittently. Repeat this exercise several times – resting for a moment or two at frequent intervals. Squeeze the eyes shut very tight – then open wide, rolling them around.

All these exercises are good when done in moderation. Preventing eye strain and dysfunction is much easier than curing them after they have become apparent.

Some simple things we can do to help our eyes in the case of referrable headaches, eye muscle problems or visual defects:

1. Holding your fingers in front of your nose, spread and wiggle the fingers.

2. Look at a large clock, follow the figures around the clock and reverse the procedure. Then do it with the eyes closed as well.

3. Place the index finger of either hand at the tip of the nose, then extend to arm's length and follow the movement with your eyes. Bring your hand to the eyes, and reverse the action.

4. Turn your face towards the sun and through closed eyelids look at the sun. Then place your hand in front of your eyes and slowly open the fingers, like a lattice work, and gaze at the sun through the fingers, opening and closing the eyelids as well as the fingers. Open and flutter the eyelids.

5. Write imaginary words with the tip of the nose. It is difficult but is beneficial and quick results can be obtained.

6. Place a piece of card in front of your face at the nose. Block out the central vision and use the peripheral vision. This makes the peripheral muscles work. In a car do the same (if you are not driving) and note the passing telegraph poles. Hold the card thus until your eyes begin to tingle, which means they are tired.

The simplicity of these exercises should not deter you from their use. I am sure that if you make a serious effort you will be surprised and pleased by how effective these simple measures can be.

17

Healthy Ears

I have heard people contemplating whether it would be worse not being able to see, or not being able to hear. It must be hoped that no one will ever be forced to make such a decision because it would be an extremely difficult choice. Not being able to see means lack of independence and missing out on some very beautiful visual experiences, while not being able to hear means isolation from conversation and communication with others, not knowing the sound of music, or listening to birdsong. I have had different answers from people who have different priorities, depending on their personal experiences.

The ears are equally as sensitive to moods and emotions as any of the other organs, and sometimes we find ourselves guilty of closing our ears because we do not want to hear what is being said. Sometimes we miss one small word and the context of the entire sentence changes. Language is the most superb means of communication, but without hearing language is relegated to written communication only. We spend very little time or attention on our ears, unless we have some physical peculiarities, such as large ears, or ears that stand out instead of lying flat against the head. However, this has no bearing on the actual ability of hearing. Ears can hardly be called an attractive feature. They do not have a romantic or sensual attraction like the skin, eyes or lips.

As I set much store by vibrations, the ears fascinate me because they react to the smallest movement or sound. A slight movement can have a frequency of 100 vibrations per second. The middle C note on a piano gives about 250 vibrations per second. One octave higher than middle C has more than 500 vibrations per second. The highest tone the human ear can detect involves some 20,000 vibrations per second. Sometimes I think that the ears, the only non-streamlined part of the human body, act like aerials. Think about it: the reason we have two eyes is so that we can have a wide panoramic view, or a telescopic view; having two ears allows us to receive stereophonic sounds. It must have been tragic for Beethoven to be struck by deafness because of otosclerosis. Many hearing problems originate because of infection in the middle ear. A minor catarrhal condition can eventually result in tinnitus, and if there is a build-up of fluid Ménière's disease can develop.

We rarely consider the fact that the ear is divided into three parts: the external ear, the middle ear and the inner ear. Each part performs an important function. The external ear consists of the auricle and ear canal. These structures gather the sound and direct it towards the eardrum membrane.

The middle ear chamber lies between the external and the inner ear. This chamber is connected to the back of the throat by way of the Eustachian tube, which serves as a pressure-equalising valve. The middle ear consists of an eardrum membrane and three small ear bones. These structures transmit sound vibrations to the inner ear, and in so doing they act as a transformer converting sound vibrations in the external ear canal into fluid waves in the inner ear. A disturbance of the Eustachian tube, eardrum membrane or the bones may result in a conductive hearing impairment.

The inner ear chamber contains the microscopic nerve endings, based in fluids. Inner ear fluid waves stimulate the delicate inner endings, which in turn transmit sound energy to the brain where it is interpreted. A disturbance in the inner ear fluids or nerve endings may result in a sensory neural hearing impairment.

The Eustachian tubes open for a fraction of a second periodically, about once every three minutes, in response to swallowing or yawning. In so doing they allow air into the middle ear to replace air that is let out. Anything that interferes with the periodic opening and closing of the Eustachian tubes may result in hearing impairment or other symptoms. This last problem I have often come across with people who have hearing problems as a result of the change in pressure from travelling by plane. If such a problem goes unchecked it can persist for many years. Very often such problems can be cleared quite successfully with cranial osteopathy. I often tell my patients about the following technique, because if it is done carefully, it need not necessarily be performed by a medically qualified person: you may do it yourself, or else enlist the gentle help of someone you trust.

A technique for hearing

The basic intention of this technique is to open the Eustachian tubes which lead from the throat to the inner ear. This will give relief to people who are suffering from head noises, tinnitus, vertigo and nausea. It is even possible for severe coughing to be relieved in this way.

Place both index fingers into the ear canals (make sure you have short fingernails), and place your thumbs over the frontal bone and the rest of the hand to the back of the skull. The technique is to simply pull towards you with your index fingers, then push away from your body direction. It is really a back and forth motion, keeping the index finger tightly in the ear canal. Try not to produce any unnecessary pain – and do not use at all in the case of an acute earache.

Dr Andrew Taylor Still, the father of osteopathy, always emphasised that for techniques to be most effective, they should be gentle, easy and scientific. It upsets me when I see anyone using a rigid object in the ears. Cotton wool will do nicely, but never use anything non-flexible. Even cotton wool buds designed for this specific purpose should be used very carefully, and never entrust this task to young children. In the case of an ear infection, as a natural antibiotic use Echinaforce twice daily (fifteen to twenty drops) or the herbal remedy Plantago (twice a day, fifteen drops before meals), which is also helpful for clearing wax from the ears. An alternative method is to sprinkle five drops of Plantago on a small piece of cotton wool, and push it deep into the ear.

The origin of deafness may be a disease, catarrh, injury or shock. Deafness can easily occur following a trauma or psychological problems, and when treating such conditions, the practitioner is well advised to investigate this aspect of a patient's life. Head noises are sometimes an indication of a catarrhal condition or high blood pressure. I recently had a patient who was badly in need of treatment for mastoiditis. The mastoid bone is situated behind the ear and directly connected with the middle and inner ear, linked with the nose, mouth and throat. Mastoiditis is inflammation of the mastoid bone and great care should always be taken in such cases because surgery is often difficult or impossible. In this case the patient was fortunate because his specialist had managed to clear the inflammation without having to resort to surgery. When the situation had settled down, however, the patient's hearing was still somewhat impaired, and he then attended my clinic for acupuncture and cranial osteopathic treatment, together with some natural remedies. During the treatment we managed to eliminate some waste matter from the ear that had been the cause of the hearing impairment, and needless to say the patient was delighted with the outcome.

We see this often with tinnitus. This condition can be the cause of major psychological problems, and I can sympathise with people who have told me that it drives them mad. Some people have become addicted to a 'Walkman' because the sound that pours into their ears all day long drowns out the noises that go on inside their head. Just imagine how awful it would be never to hear silence.

Often with tinnitus patients I detect a fungal condition in the ear and I have also noticed that such patients frequently suffer from a *Candida albicans* condition. A long-standing catarrhal condition in the inner ears may have developed into a fungal condition. Such patients should be very careful with their diet, remembering to take honey, garlic and supplementary herbal remedies, and they should also drastically reduce their salt intake. Many of my tinnitus patients have responded well to acupuncture treatment, and to the remedy *Ginkgo biloba*, which increases the blood circulation to help clear the problem. Some patients have reacted very well to some cotton wool sprinkled with five drops of *Spilanthes* pushed into the ear, and left in place overnight. Sometimes a neck manipulation is required to overcome some cervical problems, or cranial osteopathic treatment. These therapies can be of great help for tinnitus. Taking a niacin supplement may also be beneficial.

Ménière's disease is an even more difficult condition to overcome. This is a condition where the semi-circular canals of the inner ear are affected and dizziness or vertigo becomes a symptom. The treatment for Ménière's disease is not straightforward, because this is such a persistent problem. However, with some manipulatory treatment and the use of a strong natural antibiotic such as Phyto-Biotic, and the remedy Petasan, possibly combined with acupuncture, good results can be obtained. All middle ear diseases will react well to Echinaforce, Plantago and Galeopsis, and the application of cold fermentations several times daily. These fermentations should be placed on the back of the ear – not actually on the ear itself, but on the part where the ear joins the head.

From one of my nurses I learned that she had been bothered greatly by a catarrhal condition in her ear, which she had not been able to clear with prescribed drugs. She decided to follow her grandmother's advice, which was as follows: Finely chop an onion and put the onion pieces in some hot water and leave to cool slightly. Then put the onion mass, which will resemble a thick paste, in a piece of clean linen and place this compress on the ear. Cover with a towel and leave this in place for fifteen to twenty minutes. She told me that when she removed the compress waste matter could be eliminated from the ear. After this was done she felt much better: her hearing had improved and the head noises had disappeared. She also applied some gentle massage and then kept her ears clear with the remedies which I have already mentioned earlier in this chapter.

Gentle massage in the form of lymphatic drainage is considered to be beneficial and in this field Dr Vodder has devised a technique which is called 'rhythmic resistive therapy'. With this technique Dr Vodder introduced a new approach to some of the problems of structural adjustment in the physiological performance of the body tissues, and with his permission I will include below some of his explanations and his directions for treatment.

The skeleton of the extremities consists of a series of bones and their articulations, limited to movements determined by the anatomical structure of the articulating surfaces. A striated muscle attached to two or more bones by its tendonous extremities, origin and insertion, by contraction, moves the less fixed part over a greater range than it moves the more fixed bone or parts. To possess a clear concept of the values of striated muscle contraction, we must assume that the muscle contracts toward a midpoint in the muscle and obviously away from its origin and insertion.

Locomotion is only one of the many ways with which man adapts himself to his environment, through the medium of skeletal muscle contraction. The contraction of the skeletal muscles and their resultant movements explain the basic factors in every reaction to intrinsic and extrinsic influences whether it be a smile, speech, pupillary contraction and dilation, gastrointestinal peristalsis or the tiny waves that move the lymph in respiration – to name a few of the possible symptoms.

Motion through muscular action is the one outstanding expression of energy responsible for continuous activation. This implies a normal circulation of blood, fluids and the removal of waste.

The heart, the muscle-in-chief of the major functions of the body, pumps the blood to the cell. Pressure to overcome many normal obstructions is required. This responsibility belongs to the heart, but the responsibility of the muscles is to return the blood in the veins to the heart. The 'respiratory pump' activated by the respiratory muscles aids in the venous flow from the lungs to the heart. The diaphragm contraction overcomes the resistance of the uphill flow in the valveless veins of the abdomen to raise the blood to the thoracic level to the heart.

Each muscle involved in the restricted movements of a single vertebra becomes weakened through lack of motion, which is essential to its own blood supply. Tone diminishes and until the muscle is reconditioned to normal tone and contraction, the freedom of fluid flow is obstructed.

The source of energy for contraction is nutrition – that is food, water, minerals, vitamins and oxygen. The absence of sufficient amino acids results in atony and may lead to atrophy and a sequel of weakness in standing, walking and lifting, diminished respiration, heart action slowing the return of venous blood to the heart, a stasis of tissue fluids and low metabolic rate. The retention of waste, urea, carbon dioxide, creatinine and uric acid ensues, with a gradual increase of fatigue.

Dr Still stated, 'My philosophy of manipulation is based on an absolute knowledge of each and every bone in the body, their several parts in articulation, and their normal movements.' We fully realise that the motion to restore is the one outstanding force that maintains normalcy in all movable parts, particularly the fascia and the tissue, and this motion is the result of muscle contraction.

As we know, the lymph glands play a significant role in many parts of the body, but especially in the ear, nose and throat, and as the lymph system is adversely affected by the waste material that is stored, and not properly eliminated from the body, this technique is very effective. I also advise taking Oil of Evening Primrose (three 500 mg capsules, last thing at night). Usually, the lymph system is most active during the hours of sleep and this will be further stimulated by the Oil of Evening Primrose.

Vertigo and dizziness can also be caused by ear problems and often some gentle manipulation may be helpful here. Unless there is an underlying blood pressure problem I often prescribe herbal and homoeopathic remedies such as *Cocculus* and *Ginkgo biloba* (fifteen drops, three times a day). Sometimes two tablets of Kelpasan taken first thing in the morning with some warm water can also help. First of all, however, you must make sure that the vertigo condition is not a sign of high blood pressure or hypertension.

Yet again, diet plays a role and needs consideration, as all dairy foods are mucus-forming, which will not help the situation. Cut out all dairy foods except yoghurt and cottage cheese, and substitute soya milk or goat's milk. Salt is also a big enemy in these conditions and I recommend an increase in the intake of honey and garlic.

If the ear is constantly discharging I also advise taking *Hepar sulph D4*. In the case of normal earache it is preferable to use some warm St John's wort oil, placed deep into the ear. An old-fashioned method is to use almond oil, but be careful not to overdo this treatment. The correct method is to heat the spoon, so making the temperature of the oil more pleasant for the ear. I prefer, however, to use aromatherapy oils or inhale the vapours of these oils. Aromatherapy can be of great help for these conditions.

With real hearing loss and possible deafness acupuncture may help to heal the affected nerve. I remember reading a newspaper article on this subject which caused me some concern. This article featured an interview with a patient of mine, who had been almost deaf when he first attended my clinic, and in the interviews he claimed that the acupuncture treatment he received had cured his deafness. I was concerned because his deafness had indeed diminished, but it had not been cured. Also, the other remedies I had prescribed had contributed to his partial recovery. Hearing deficiencies or ear inflammations can be overcome, but these problems are not to be taken lightly, and proper medical advice should be sought. Sometimes complementary medicine can play a big role alongside orthodox medicine, and this is especially true in the case of ear problems. The major factors are to control congestion and to maintain a positive outlook and determination to help yourself.

18

A Healthy Nose

When we were young, my grandmother used to tell us not to touch our nose with our fingers, because the lips and nose are highly sensitive to any infections. The respiratory organs comprise the nose, the trachea and the lungs. As with the ears, most people are more aware of the shape of their nose than of its function. It may be too big or too small, or bent, and some people who are unhappy with the shape decide to rectify it by way of plastic surgery. However, the proper function of the nose is of far greater importance than its aesthetic appearance. This miraculously planned small part of the anatomy has a very important function. We are taught to breathe always through the nose and not through the mouth, as the nose filters any bacteria and dust from the intake of air. Indeed, we must be careful not to breathe through the mouth, because the screening device in the nose will protect us from infection and colds, and therefore help the bronchial passages and the lungs to stay healthy.

The nose will react to any sensation of smell, and perhaps it is only when this ability has become impaired, that we fully appreciate how useful and pleasant this sense is. We have to learn how to inhale properly and breathing through the nose should take place without hindrance or effort. Often this function becomes more laborious in cases of enlarged adenoids and infection of the mucous membranes. When this free breathing is obstructed and the nasal passages or bronchi become swollen, a person will begin to snore, and any swelling in the adenoids or the nose should always be corrected. For this purpose the herbal remedy *Marum verum* is useful (fifteen drops, taken three times a day), or you should inhale some of the very useful aromatherapy oils. Alternatively, adding a few drops of PoHo oil to a bowl of warm water, covering the bowl and head with a towel and so gently inhaling these aromatic vapours, can also clear the passages. In some cases tea-tree oil will help to clear the watery discharge from the nose and remove some of the built up catarrh. It is always wonderful when the sense of smell returns, after having temporarily lost it.

The nose can be divided in two halves and it is very rich in blood vessels, nerves and glands. The microscopic cells, called silia, are attuned to the rhythmic movement of the nose. Therefore it is worth while to know that nose exercises can help in its function. The mucous membranes which are located in the upper nose have between ten and twenty million cells. It is those cells that enable us to smell, and each cell has a receptor for a specialised nerve cell.

The sensory hairs – called the retio-respiratoria – provide protection and play a role in the breathing process. These are on either side of the nose promontory and it is almost unbelievable to think that in such a small part of the body there are ten to twelve million of these little hairs whose function is to locate the correct smell.

It is interesting to see how this faculty varies according to sex, because men appear to be much more sensitive to smell than women, which helps to explain why nuanceurs, who work in the perfume industry, are mostly men, while it is predominantly women who tend to wear perfume. With animals we only need to think of police dogs or sniffer dogs, who have such a well-developed sense of smell.

The message sent to the brain by our sense of smell is quite extraordinary. If we know how the nose works, we should not be surprised at how many allergies there are which directly affect this organ. Allergic conditions such as hay fever need to be checked from the very beginning in order to try and keep them under control and avoid their very uncomfortable side-effects.

When we consider allergies, we see the influence of air on the nose and throat. Inhaling different substances can cause the eyes to itch and run, block the nose, make us sneeze and wheeze and often develop a cough. In hay fever, when the pollen count in the air is rising, this is exactly what happens. The tiny particles of pollen that are carried in the air can cause the most dramatic symptoms. Unless one protects oneself problems of gigantic proportions can result.

Pollinosan is a homoeopathic remedy especially designed for treating hay fever and allergic conditions. It not only protects against allergens and irritants but it also desensitises the system. With regard to diet, people who are prone to hay fever should avoid dairy foods and drastically reduce their intake of salt. When the nose is blocked with catarrh it needs treatment immediately. Not only hay fever, but infections or inflammations such as sinusitis can be most uncomfortable. The preferred treatment for sinusitis is acupuncture, soft-tissue massage and the remedies Sinu-Check and SNS Formula.

Polyps in the nose affect the mucous membranes and catarrhal conditions caused by polyps can be very unpleasant. It is possible to relieve the mucous membranes by sniffing ice-cold water with a few drops of lemon juice added to it. Taking *Marum verum* (three times a day, ten drops before meals), and Petasan (three times a day, ten drops after meals), is usually beneficial. When properly treated these ailments need not rule our lives.

The other day I had to advise a lady who had had a fracture of the nose to see a specialist. Not only was her breathing laboured, but she had developed a condition called rhinitis, which was obstructing her breathing. I advised her to inhale steam with either tea-tree oil or PoHo oil, and to use Sinu-Check and SNS Formula together. This provided some relief, but the damage inflicted by the fracture was too severe, and surgery was esssential. She came to see me afterwards and she felt herself to blame because she had let the condition deteriorate until it was almost too late to have it corrected.

Sometimes we see that a minor obstruction, that could have been easily solved in infancy, can cause breathing problems if left untreated, sometimes developing into asthmatic or bronchial problems. It is very important that these patients are able to breathe freely.

Nasal irrigation is a commonly used method to clear nasal congestion. Preparations for nasal irrigation should consist of salt, bicarbonate of soda and boric acid (in the proportions 3 : 2 : 1). Allow one teaspoon of this mixture to one pint of water at a temperature of 110 °F. Prepare a quart of this mixture in a suitable container and use a slightly lubricated rubber catheter. If preferred, a simple saline solution can be used and here the proportion should be one level teaspoon of salt to one pint of hot water.

At your request your chemist will make up the following combination fluid, which may be used after the nasal irrigation and can be easily applied with the help of an atomiser spray:

Menthol	10 grains
Camphor	30 grains
Oil of Eucalyptus	1 dram
Thymol	1 dram

It should be remembered that with simple nasal irrigation more serious conditions such as rhinitis, sinusitis or other nasal problems can be avoided. To give you a better understanding of the sinus function you should know that the sinuses connect directly or indirectly with the nasal cavity. Bearing in mind the existence of the three bodies of man, the physical, mental and emotional bodies, it is significant to note that sinuses receive the breath of life directly and unmodified, as it flows from the universe, through the nose and before any other organs have a chance to select and absorb any substance.

The sinuses are lined with mucous membranes extending from the nose. Therefore all disorders that affect the nose will rapidly spread to the sinuses. The nose is the first organ that reacts to polluted air and that reaction we recognise as a cold. The inflammation resulting from the effect of polluted air extends from the nasal mucous lining to the sinuses, causing such disorders as frontal headache (frontal sinus), pain in the cheek (maxillary sinus), pain between the eyes (ethmoidal sinus) and deep-seated pain in the back of the eyes (sphenoidal sinus). Trouble starts when the mucous excretions of the lining of the maxillary sinus, in inflammatory conditions, fill up this sinus as the opening is at the upper part.

It has been stated that the five physical senses of conscious man are the externalised products of the five corresponding spiritual centres, which are as follows:

1. Frontal sinus: a cavity in the frontal bone of the skull
2. Sphenoidal sinus: a cavity in the sphenoid bone of the skull
3. Maxillary sinus: the largest of the five and resembling a pyramid in shape
4. Palatine sinus: a cavity in the orbital process of the palatine bone and opening into either the sphenoidal or posterior ethmoidal sinus
5. Ethmoidal sinus: this chamber consisting of numerous cavities occupying the labyrinth of the ethmoidal bone and housing the small mysterious glands known as the intellectual organs

These sinuses, or air centres, and the small glands contained in them, constitute the spiritual sense centres that receive the higher intelligence, which is too subtle for contact by the five physical senses of conscious man. Into these chambers or sinuses flows a peculiar gaseous substance, known to the Ancients as the mental spirit. The small glands – the intellectual organs – located in the skull near the point where the nose joins the forehead, are activated by the mental spirit that passes through the nostrils into the ordinate and collaborate with the sinuses. This is the chief spiritual centre of man.

Polluted air damages the sinuses and thus the power of resisting disease is weakened and the power of attaining intuitive powers is also diminished.

These chambers are in direct contact with the pineal and pituitary glands belonging to the endocrine system, which are also of a psychic nature and influential sections of the universal mind. Herein lies the means to release any disease through cranial adjustments that will break up harmful formations in these chambers.

From the above we see again how significant a role these three bodies of man play in nasal conditions. Unfortunately, the human motor is rarely allowed to change into a lower gear and peaceful intervals these days are few and far between. Today, our business and private life is ruled by frustration, major and minor irritations and a subsequent magnification of the emotions of fear, anger, anxiety and insecurity.

Thousands of years ago, this energy control mechanism was of the greatest importance for survival. Today, conditions which imposed this fight or flight syndrome are not required. Instead, what is needed is self-control, common sense and quiet thinking along rational lines. Nevertheless, man's body is the same as it was thousands of years ago, and this primitive combat instinct remains within it. However, modern civilisation will not interfere if only he can learn to control this energy-expending mechanism of the body. The answer to this is to follow in the footsteps of our ancestors, whose knowledge was intuitive: the diet should be high in carbohydrates and low in protein.

Every human body possesses fighting equipment that enables it to organise aggressive action, but this action was intended to be only temporary. Our modern environment has made it permanent. What happens to us in our modern environment, that is sadly so utterly divorced from natural law? When the sympathetic division of the autonomic nervous system is organised to arouse the body for aggressive action, other vital changes take place in the body. The sympathetic division controls the alkalinity of the blood so that when it is activated there is an increase in the blood alkaline level. This is quite in order under extraordinary circumstances, but becomes detrimental when allowed to continue on a daily basis.

There is a gradual change from the normally healthy acid/alkaline balance reaction of the urine to alkaline. This increased alkalinity precipitates free calcium on the walls of the body cells so that the permeability of the cell wall decreases, preventing vital food materials and oxygen from entering. The cell factory, which produces heat, energy, carbonic acid, lactic acid, phosphoric and sulphuric acid, then shuts down. Thus the action of the energy-producing mechanism, the sympathetic divider of the autonomic nervous system and adrenal glands, cuts off the vital activity of the body cells. It is no longer an emergency arousal but a permanent high-gear performance that is needed to cope with a stress induced by modern life. No wonder coronary thrombosis and cancer are on the increase.

Of the many factors inducing this are denatured foods, processed foods, alcohol, drugs, smoking, prolonged physical and mental work, producing in their turn emotional frustrations and fears.

Food grown in cold climates will calm down an over-active sympathetic division, whilst food grown in warmer zones will stimulate this division. Thus, by means of proper food intake, nature seeks to maintain a working balance between the two divisions of the autonomic nervous system.

An acidic reaction of the urine indicates that osmotic pressure in the blood and hydrochloric stomach secretion are normal, and that the sympathetic nervous division is under control. The human motor is then in low gear. Furthermore, the parasympathetic division which builds and stores the body's reserves, will be in control.

Coming back to our increased alkalinity and clogging of the body cells, thus preventing the vital food material and oxygen from entering: this produces a short circuit within the affected portion of the body. The life force is momentarily cut off, as it were, from the furthermost negative pole in the pelvic basin to that of the positive in the brain. Sickness, pain and disease are the result.

To restore normality, just as one would restore a portion of the lighting system in the house, both ends of the positive and negative poles of the sympathetic and parasympathetic nervous system must be similarly restored so that the life-giving force may circulate once again.

All involuntary spasms, tensions and contractures of the body are neutralised and restored to normality when this is accomplished, and the body automatically shifts into low gear as ordained by nature. When it is fully realised that these body currents or energy fields are prevented from flowing by obstructions or short circuits through a lack of polarity potential, the principle can be understood more clearly by the practitioner.

Fear, emotional upset, day-to-day frustrations and other inhibitions, have been observed to produce an alkaline urine reaction in individuals. A simple acute anxiety neurosis will produce this. This continued alkalinity will, in time, produce an environment that is conducive to the invasion of bacteria. Bacteria cannot thrive in an acid medium. This problem will be compounded by a faulty diet, producing an alkalinity of the blood. A natural low-protein and high-carbohydrate diet recommended by nature, organises the body for peace and quiet, enabling it to build up and store reserves to be used in times of need. But when man rearranges nature's plans to suit his own desires, placing more emphasis on protein instead of carbohydrates in his diet, he is organising his body for continual fight and flight, as did his ancestors in the cave.

If people live under conditions which arouse the negative emotions described above, and eat this high-protein and low-carbohydrate diet, the brain, muscular system, digestive tracts and nervous system will all be affected and the entire body will suffer.

The manual stimulation technique often referred to as the spheno-palatine ganglion technique, is highly effective in the psychosomatic field. All emotions, stresses and tensions induced by dietary shortcomings and negative thinking with fear as its basis, is catered for, by this method.

A triangle is formed by the two sympathetic ganglia and the point of attachment and this is similar to a blown fuse between these dual polarities and the human energy field. This triangle concept was born of nature. Therefore there is what is known as the law of the triangle in the composition of matter and the manifestation of either cosmic or human energy. Snow, ice, mineral and acid crystals are all part of this adherence to nature's law of the triangle. Moreover, the triangle is one of the most ancient geometrical forms, which symbolised perfection; two points of a triangle represent the dual forces of the universe, while the third point represents perfection.

Mention should also be made of the emotional state of man and its effect upon the physical body through the sympathetic nervous system. This is symbolic of the two interlaced triangles – also the symbol of perfection of the microcosmic and macrocosmic worlds, i.e. perfection in the physical universe and the spiritual world. The six-pointed star is the symbol of the unity of both phases of existence of which man is intuitively aware, but whose senses have been blunted by material desire over the centuries.

The above is a profound explanation of the manual stimulation of the positive and negative sympathetic nerve ganglia, with further manual contact on the area affected or break in the human polar energy field, with its ultimate restorative power and thus signifying the eternal triangle in nature. It is therefore important to restore and maintain harmony restored between the ears, nose and throat to ensure that the physical, mental and emotional bodies are properly attuned.

19

A Healthy Throat

Many years ago, when I worked in China, I was taught tongue diagnosis. Much can be learned from the tongue, especially when one practises acupuncture. The tongue tells us much of what goes on inside the body, and the older generation of doctors, who were skilled at tongue diagnosis, knew exactly what to look for. The tongue will tell us a great deal about the patient's general condition, and a doctor can draw his own conclusions from possible tongue eruptions, a furry tongue, a candida tongue, or the colour of the tongue. Last time I was in China, the professor under whom I had studied previously, insisted that this time he would instruct me in throat diagnosis. The Chinese rightly believe that the throat is turning into a cesspool of bacteria, and that there are many hidden infections in the throat that have to be cleared before we can successfully treat a patient. Dr Vogel used to say in his lectures that we should disinfect the throat regularly and recommended that Molkosan be used for this purpose. Molkosan is a liquid derived from fresh whey by a natural fermentation process. It contains all the important minerals found in fresh whey such as magnesium, potassium and calcium, in concentrated form. This product is rich in natural dextrorotatory L(+) lactic acid, which in health-oriented nutrition as well as natural healing methods has a special significance. As whey is the leftover from the cheese-making process, it contains strong antiseptic characteristics, and as such is widely recommended for the treatment of athlete's foot, verrucas and warts. Half a teaspoon of Molkosan, taken in some water, mineral water, or fruit juice, twice a day, makes a refreshing drink with excellent health-promoting properties. Not only is Molkosan very good as an antiseptic, it is also excellent for the digestive system.

As useful as tongue diagnosis is, I have found throat diagnosis to be equally so. In my research project on rheumatism and arthritis, I have often seen that when the throat was cleared, so did some of the arthritic or rheumatic problems.

I need not tell you how sensitive the throat is because no matter how healthy we are, we have all in our time suffered from a sore throat. What is not widely known is that amalgam dental fillings can be the cause of a variety of obscure health problems, and therefore I frequently advise patients to have their amalgam fillings removed and replaced by composite fillings. Prior to this removal process the patient should take plenty of Molkosan and Echinaforce, for their antiseptic and antibiotic properties. Sometimes very strong detoxifiers like CPS or Chem-Ex are used to assist in this process.

I recommended these two remedies when I was consulted by a well-known patient. I remember, looking out of the window of my clinic in the Netherlands and seeing this person arrive, escorted by two aides and looking very sad. When my assistant came to inform me of his arrival, I wondered why this widely known figure had seen fit to visit my clinic. He candidly answered my questions and I learned that after a course of dental treatment some time ago he felt some kind of obstruction in his throat. He returned to the dentist and was given some liquid to gargle. When this obstruction did not clear, the dentist checked and told him not to worry because there was nothing untoward in the throat. He then visited his doctor, who also tried to reassure him that there was nothing wrong with his throat. After a number of months, at his request, the doctor checked his throat a second time and again he reported that there was nothing wrong. However, he agreed to refer the patient to a neurologist. A further check-up followed, but the neurologist also told him that his throat was clear. Some time passed and the gentleman was still concerned about an irregularity in his throat. He returned to the neurologist, who eventually referred him to a psychiatrist. This specialist, in turn, told him that there was nothing wrong with his brain, and he returned yet again to the neurologist. More studies and tests were done and, unfortunately, it eventually became clear that he had an inoperable tumour in the throat.

I listened to this story and sympathised with him. From facial diagnosis I realised that he had liver problems and that his entire system was affected. The tumour was inoperable, but when I did some tests I found signs of heavy metal. I remembered his account of the visit to the dentist, and I thought that this metal deposit might be due to amalgam. I spoke to his physician, who was willing to arrange for some hospital tests. The conclusion was that amalgam poisoning was a possibility. I immediately started on a course of treatment, as the report had suggested that a minute piece of amalgam had possibly been swallowed. This tiny piece of amalgam had worked its way into the tissue and started an infection in one of the glands, and this infection had subsequently become cancerous. The doctor in question asked me to visit this gentleman and I prescribed several detoxifying remedies, i.e. Petasan and *Viscum album*, as well as some supplementary vitamin C. To our great surprise, the small piece of amalgam, which had registered as heavy metal in my tests, dissolved and the immune system, having been boosted with the treatment, then assisted in combating the cancer process. The fight between the healthy cells and the cancerous cells was won by the influence of the immune system in overcoming the cancerous cells. Fortunately, a healthy diet combined with the above-mentioned remedies mentioned helped to fully restore the action of his liver and his condition steadily improved. The final outcome of it all was that my wife and I were invited to a special dinner as the guests of this gentleman, who is fully recovered and again able to fulfil the considerable demands of his profession.

I agree that this is one of the most extreme cases I have come across in my practice, and I was delighted to have been able to help this very pleasant gentleman to overcome this major health threat. Often when I see what is termed an incurable disease, this experience gives me the courage to go on and never give in, because complementary medicine can sometimes help in serious problems where all else has failed.

The throat can be affected by so many things. Just think of the changes in the medical approach over the last few decades. From about 1920 there was a strong belief that the tonsils – the almond-shaped bodies situated on either side of the throat, or the pharynx – should be removed because they served no purpose at all. They were merely thought to be useless appendages, which became bothersome when infected. This is totally mistaken, because the tonsils are great protectors, and it was totally overlooked that once these have been removed there is nothing anyone can do to reverse the decision. I remember when, shortly after the Second World War, tonsillectomies were performed as a matter of routine on primary school children. Sadly, this was often unnecessary. Nowadays we encounter so many problems in the throat, e.g. tonsillitis and pharyngitis, and I believe that this increase is caused by a reduced resistance to bacteria. Tonsillitis, which is an acute inflammation of the tonsils, is the result of a toxic condition. This is fairly common among people who suffer from constipation, and therefore my grandmother's advice to use castor oil occasionally to encourage the body to eliminate waste matter was not a bad idea. Tonsillitis patients are advised to gargle with diluted Molkosan and, because thorough cleansing should be undertaken, I sometimes advise patients to use the Rasayana Cleansing Course. With an acute sore throat it is often best to drink nothing but water.

I was amazed when a well-known broadcaster told me that she never ate or drank anything before a broadcast in order to keep her throat clear. This is indeed correct according to the naturopathic principle of fasting and drinking only water to keep a throat clear. The only other drinks that are permitted are herbal teas, such as chamomile or peppermint tea. A hot bicarbonate of soda or Epsom salts bath is very good in the case of tonsillitis. Cranberry or pineapple juice is also useful in cases of chronic throat problems.

I have treated quite a number of singers and found that the treatment required was often no more than some minor cranial manipulation.

Pharyngitis is another big problem I often come across, and this is symptomatic of an inflammation of the mucous membrane of the throat, affecting the voice and often lending an unusual huskiness to the voice. This problem is mostly caused by chronic bowel problems and constipation should be avoided as this will aggravate the problem. Should there be a recurrence of pharyngitis, fasting will help, or warm and cold baths. When the most acute symptoms are past a fresh fruit diet should be followed.

In cases of angina it is necessary to check for toxins and there may be a need for *Lachesis D12*, which is basically an extract of snake venom. This will be very helpful in shrinking swollen tonsils. If this remedy is taken for swollen tonsils it may avert the need for a tonsillectomy.

Externally, a cabbage leaf may be used as a poultice over the throat, held in place overnight by a scarf, allowing it to become very warm. This old-fashioned, but effective, method is often very helpful. Golden Grass Tea also will provide relief.

Public speakers who rely heavily on their voice sometimes experience the growth of polyps on their vocal chords, which causes them great inconvenience. This condition is further aggravated by cigarette smoke and in this case the best remedy is Irish moss, and therefore the Usneasan or Bronchosan preparations, which include this as an ingredient, have always been of great help.

Laryngitis can be caused by bronchitis, pneumonia, influenza, diphtheria, and excessive cigarette smoke and the inhalation of certain irritants. This condition can linger for a long time if it goes unchecked. The above-mentioned remedies also apply in such cases.

As we are talking about the tongue and the throat in this chapter we should look at the ever-growing problem of pyorrhoea, a disease of the teeth sockets and one that is very prevalent today. The roots of the teeth are affected and we see a loosening and a shrinkage of the gums. The symptoms of gingivitis are similar to pyorrhoea and in both cases diet is important and it is advisable to cleanse the teeth morning and night with a little lemon juice. Whenever I lecture alongside my friend Leonard Mervyn, from whom I have learned so much over the years, I am always happy to hear him praise the remedy Co-Enzyme Q10 for just these problems. Co-Enzyme Q10, or Ubiquinone (meaning 'everywhere'), is a normal and essential component of the mitochondria. Hence the co-enzyme is essential for the health of all human tissues and organs. It is a vitamin-like substance which is manufactured by the body; it can also be found in some foods, but seems difficult to extract from them. A food supplement of CoQ10 may be useful to ensure that there is an ample supply of this important co-factor in the tissues at all times. The mito-chondria are the energy generators of the cells and the highest proportion are found in the cells that do the most work, notably the liver, muscle tissue and the heart. Research is still ongoing to uncover the full extent of CoQ10's role in the metabolism, but leading scientists believe that it is in effect a 'biochemical spark' that releases energy from food. CoQ10 is therefore involved when we exert any physical energy. Studies have shown that obese people have lower levels of CoQ10 in their tissue cells than those who are slim. I have also successfully prescribed this remedy for a quinsy throat, a very painful condition, where there is an abscess on a tonsil. In such cases CoQ10 together with a Molkosan mouthwash is most effective.

For tonsillitis, chills or colds in the larynx, or even an infected lymph gland in the neck, there are some simple but useful manipulation techniques that can be applied. The painful side is the contact side. Place the index finger under the angle of the jaw into the neck tissues. The rest of the hand is spread out to support the head. The only movement concerns the index finger, which is moved back and forth over the area of the affected tissues. The pressure should be light at first, increasing as the pain disappears.

A further massage technique is specifically used in the case of enlarged tonsils, even though they may not necessarily be caused by infections. Massage the tonsil tissue by inserting the forefinger, which is covered by a finger cot, down the side of the mouth until past the anterior pillar. Starting with the superior pole, massage downward three or four times with firm pressure – then squeeze the tonsil from the front to the back and from the back to the front two or three times. Then proceed to the inferior pole, or base – press upward two or three times. This constitutes a treatment for one side – now use the same technique for the other side.

For young children and those that are reluctant to put their fingers in their throats, this technique is best done with tonsil suction treatment.

Massage techniques for loosening and raising the glands of the neck vary according to the gland, i.e. the parathyroid, thyroid or thymus. The parathyroid gland encapsulates two small glands on each side of the neck on the lower border of the thyroid gland, and is responsible for the calcium phosphate balance, maintaining calcium in the bones. Its function is to aid the adrenal glands by increasing the level of calcium in the bones, and to neutralise the toxic waste in the intestines.

Place the fingers of one hand between the trachea and gland – press firmly – sliding the finger up and down. Adhesions can be felt as strings or cord-like nodules, sometimes in bunches. Press the fingers in under the trachea, lifting upward and out. The thumb on the opposite side of the neck gives support only. Use the same finger technique for the opposite side of the neck.

Many years ago I accompanied my friend Dr Victor Penzer to Oxford University for a lecture on mercury amalgam toxicity. In 1985 I wrote a book on multiple sclerosis and even then I warned about the dangers of allergies to mercury amalgam, and also about the potential toxic effects of amalgam. Over the years these theories have been confirmed, and although it may remain controversial as far as dentists are concerned, we have begun to accept that this substitute in the teeth has caused more damage than could have been imagined. I always remember how Victor Penzer tried to get this message across, but it was rejected out of hand. Nowadays this knowledge is much more widely accepted, and often, when I come across these fillings affecting the mouth, throat and body as a whole, I have had to advise patients to enquire whether their dentist is prepared to reverse the situation. My own dentist has kindly replaced my amalgam fillings with composite fillings and his comments afterwards were that not only had the appearance of my teeth improved, but that my body would benefit.

The war still goes on and I have tried for years to get the message across because I have seen for myself the effects of amalgam fillings on many patients. I can only advise that these patients ask their dentist to reverse the situation. Tests show that the silver mercury in the teeth inactivates enzymes and possibly even the hormonal system. It has been shown that this could be a possible cause of any of the following conditions: excess lactic acid production, muscular physiology problems, damage to the heart tissue, insulin disturbance, red blood cell interference possibly resulting in anaemia, and a host of other problems that have been noted in the findings of many practitioners. Even back in the nineteenth century the American Society of Dental Surgeons required its members to sign a written agreement not to put amalgam fillings in patients' mouths. In 1972 a Dr Brian Hellewel warned Dr David Owen, then a cabinet minister in the Labour government, that in the face of the mounting evidence of danger, and the absence of evidence of safety, it was his duty to advise him that the use of mercury dental amalgam for fillings in the teeth of pregnant women should be discontinued.

As this is a chapter on the throat I will go no further into this subject, but people should be aware of the dangers posed by this practice, and for those who wish to know more, there are quite a number of publications devoted to this subject in much more detail. At the best of times, our teeth are a reflection of many body functions. Dental conditions can affect the heart, stomach, liver, endocrine system, circulation, ears, nose and throat. I remember hearing about Dr Issels, a German practitioner of complementary medicine, who became well known because of his unorthodox treatment of cancer patients. If he had a seriously ill patient, he had his patients' teeth removed. This I considered extremely drastic, but knowing the results of recent research, I can now appreciate that he wanted to protect his patients from hidden infections of the teeth and from the influence of dental fillings on their general health.

Good dental care will also influence the throat. The salivary glands, which lie in the throat, produce the necessary saliva – about 1.5 litres in a period of twenty-four hours. These glands should be encouraged to fulfil their task without placing obstructions in their way. It is very important to realise that saliva is essential for life. It is formed in the salivary glands, to enable speech, to aid digestion by good mastication, and with the amylase enzyme it forms a barrier against bacteria. It not only functions as an anti-microbe agent, but it cleanses by acting as a barrier, aids digestion, and protects the mucous membranes.

People with a dry mouth and throat, caused by insufficient saliva production, will experience problems with speaking, chewing and swallowing and also frequently lose their sense of taste. These functional problems will also influence the teeth. If we look at the physical, mental and emotional bodies, the primary causes of a dry mouth include emotion, worry, fear, depression, stress, neurosis – and anti-histamines. Most problems of this type occur in the saliva centre. Other causes are encephalitis, tumours, operations, diuretics and anti-depressants. The factors that influence the saliva glands are obstructions, infections, tumours and chemotherapy and radiation therapy. Factors that influence the electrolytes of the fluid balance are dehydration, haemorrhage, diabetes, insufficient heart function, oedema, uraemia, hypertension, thyroid dysfunction, hormonal imbalances, Parkinson's disease, anaemia and diuretics. Therefore we can see clearly that a detrimental influence on any of the three bodies will lead to problems. In osteopathy we also see this imbalance as structural. In some conditions we have to perform a TMJ application. This technique is an application of the temporo-mandibular joint (TMJ) adjustment. Not only should the teeth of the upper and lower jaws fit well together, because headaches could otherwise result, but disalignment can also cause problems with the gums, muscles and bones. In lectures to dentists I often mention this because I know that this problem occurs in one in four people. Unfortunately, the TMJ is often out of alignment and this can have all kinds of repercussions, such as toothache, loose and broken teeth, headaches and even sciatica because it affects so many parts of the body.

I saw this quite clearly in the case of a well-known singer who came to me for treatment. I had heard her sing in concerts and I was a great admirer, but she was in despair when she visited my clinic, because she was experiencing problems with her voice. As soon as I saw her I realised that she had a jaw problem that required adjustment. Years ago, I was instructed by a famous chiropractor in the USA, named Dr Gonstead, and with the help of his teachings I have been able to successfully treat many people. I was absolutely shattered when I read an information sheet that this patient had been given by the hospital. It stated that, indeed, the temporo-mandibular dysfunction does cause problems for many people. What I could hardly believe was that these patients were fitted with a splint that was to be worn at all times with the exception of mealtimes and while brushing their teeth. The patient had to keep a daily record while wearing this splint – a period of twelve weeks. If there was no significant improvement, another treatment with an alternative splint would be offered, either a possible splint adjustment or a further investigation. If the symptoms had been alleviated after twelve weeks the advice was to wear the splint at night time only.

A qualified osteopath or chiropractor is able to effect the required adjustment in a matter of minutes, unless there is bone deterioration or arthritis, in which case the treatment may be somewhat more complicated. You can imagine my disbelief that, in 1995, treatment with splints for periods of up to twelve weeks still existed, while the patient could have been helped in a matter of minutes. I am happy to say that this singer was absolutely well again after a single treatment session. The problem was that because of the jaw dislocation, the hyoid or lingual bone, which has an important structural functional relation with the tongue, larynx and pharynx, was slightly damaged. Acute and chronic infections that cause voice impairment commonly result from lesions of this bone. Such lesions may be caused by the inflammation and contracture of one or more of several muscle groups: the sterno-hyoid, thyro-hyoid and omo-hyoid groups, with their several fascias and apro-neuroses. This bone can be fractured by trauma, including careless treatment, sometimes by a dentist, and while it will eventually heal, it causes plenty of discomfort and pain. For this reason I have developed a safe and effective treatment, which has also been very helpful in cases of catarrh, sinusitis and related conditions.

A constant cough, coming from deep within the chest, should also be investigated. When this condition is persistent, investigation may indicate that the underlying cause is psychological or emotional. When there is stress or emotional turmoil, the outcome is often toxicity. Toxins in the body will affect our overall health in many ways, and require a detoxification process. Irritation or aggression, when we clench the teeth or place the tongue between the teeth, can impair the speech or render it impossible. These emotions can be subdued, and yet they can contribute to a throat or speech problem, because the original complaint remains untreated or unnoticed. Think of the expression 'I had a lump in my throat'. This commonly happens to people who are required to speak in public, until suddenly they no longer feel able to do so. They become nervous and upset, and because of this tension a great deal of pressure and tightness is exerted on every muscle and bone, so that speaking becomes almost impossible. Another effect is sickness or an inability to eat. The throat may become inflamed, possibly affecting the thyroid, which in turn will affect the entire endocrine system, making it even more tense, so that the entire body experiences tension. Be very gentle with yourself, especially when dealing with life's experiences with all their emotions of fear, worry, hatred and misunderstanding. Try to replace the negative with the positive. Think again of the three monkeys: 'Hear no evil, see no evil and speak no evil.' The throat has a tremendous influence on the emotional body and it responds very favourably to the universal law that with love we can overcome everything.

20

A Healthy Skin

In previous chapters I have tried to point out that when building our house of health, we should know what goes on inside. We have dealt with many parts of the body and now we will look at the outside of the house. We are usually more concerned with the outside than with the inside. But from the inside of the body the outside is born. Remember the three principles I follow in reaching a diagnosis: to look, listen and feel. Outwardly, the body tells us many things, not only by way of facial diagnosis and with the help of iridology, but also through the skin. In order to produce a healthy skin, the inside must be healthy. For example, a yellow skin indicates liver problems, and dark circles under the eyes point to kidney problems. A clammy hand will tell us that the kidneys need cleansing. 'A healthy mind in a healthy body', so the saying goes, and a healthy skin is the outward sign of a healthy body. The outside should be as healthy as possible and we will know that the inside will be all right too.

When looking at the skin we should be aware that a healthy diet, good personal hygiene and a spirit of relaxation count as the most important ingredients to help the skin and its complexion. Julius Caesar was very concerned about his hair loss, and Cleopatra bathed in asses' milk to retain the youthful lustre and elasticity of her skin. The skin is the largest organ of the body and, apart from the stomach, it has its own effective forms of protection. Normal perspiration and breathing in and out maintain the moisture of the skin. Heat will help the skin, and its many glands keep it supple. A bruise or a cut shows how quickly the skin recovers from injury.

Eczema or dermatitis patients sometimes scratch themselves until the skin is damaged. The use of strong acid creams or soaps can make the skin very sensitive and can cause considerable problems. Clothing is another source of problems: some people cannot bear to wear anything made with artificial fibres, and this poses a problem for many people. Certain chemicals, and even metals such as copper, nickel, gold or silver, can also cause skin problems. Even a pair of plastic spectacles or an artificial tooth can cause skin irritations. Therefore in the case of allergic reactions the body may need to be desensitised, and the cause of an allergic reaction may be hard to pinpoint. I remember years ago, when I was still involved in pharmaceuticals, we were shocked to learn that a well-known cosmetics manufacturer had to withdraw an entire lipstick range from the market because it was a major irritant and was suspected of being a possible source of cancer. In the use of cosmetics, please always make very sure that they do not contain any harmful ingredients. Do not take any risks, and always buy cosmetic products from producers that are known to be responsible about the contents of their products. Hair colourings also often cause dermatitis and undefined scalp irritations. Furthermore, we must not forget that our skin also comes into contact with these substances and these can have a carcinogenic effect. Skin cancer was very common among chimney sweeps. Other people, who have spent their working lives in the chemical industry, have experienced health problems as a result and burns in particular can have a drastic effect on the skin. I have already said that the skin often shows what goes on inside, and therefore lumps or a rash can be a signal of internal problems. In the swimming pool or sauna we can easily contract a verruca or a fungal infection. A metal identity plate can be the cause of an irritation, or even the metal backing of a wrist watch. Certain plants or herbs can cause a skin eruption. Even the smallest interference with the skin, such as an allergy, can lead to drastic problems. Skin problems may occur after being angry, emotionally upset, going through physical or mental trauma, or as the result of a physical illness such as shingles. It is essential that we look at all aspects when trying to trace the possible cause.

I am reminded of the mother who brought her teenage daughter to me who was afflicted with a nasty skin condition. The girl indeed was a sorry sight and the mother told me that she had arranged all possible tests for her daughter, among them a hair test, a blood test and a skin test. Several offenders in her diet had been isolated. She had already taken her daughter to three different specialists and money was no object. However, she had taken their advice and started to eliminate all the foods that each test had shown the girl to be allergic to. The sorry outcome was that this girl was suffering from scurvy, because the mother had eliminated too many food items from the girl's diet. This was shocking. The mother had paid a fortune for all these tests, and had completely overlooked the fact that the child required vitamins and minerals, and the result was that I could diagnose nothing other than scurvy caused by malnutrition.

Once the real allergy was diagnosed and I had desensitised the girl with some specific remedies, such as *Harpagophytum*, *Viola tricolor*, Evening

Primrose and Echinaforce, her skin improved immediately. I also prescribed extra supplements of vitamin C, and the scurvy condition was soon brought under control. Allergy tests are very important, and I am often asked about my treatment methods. Usually my answer is that I do not specifically treat the allergies themselves, but I strengthen the immune system. It is inexplicable, but one day one can be allergic to wheat, and a few days later this is no longer the case, but then suddenly there may be an allergy to milk, dust, or anything else for that matter. The immune system changes with every tick of the clock, and only once I have built up the immune system and if the skin problem still occurs, will I then undertake allergy tests. Such was the case with a gentle young girl with a suppurating skin disease, which had so far remained unidentified by the doctors and dermatologists she had seen. I felt a bit like Sherlock Holmes in the process of finding out the problem. She assured me that her diet was very healthy and she talked me through all she would eat in a day, when I accidentally discovered that she was allergic to bananas. This girl still eats bananas, but her mistake was that each morning she would have a healthy breakfast of muesli with fresh fruits. However, the banana is a jealous fruit, as is the melon, and I always advise that these should be eaten on their own. The same advice applies to vegetables and fruit, which should never be eaten together. It is much better to eat them separately, because the digestive system cannot always cope and then an allergic reaction can easily occur.

Wheat allergies are the order of the day and I think that this is basically because of the modern techniques used for growing wheat. I remember a gentleman who had travelled a long distance to my clinic. He was a market-gardener, specialising in lettuces. He was very successful at what he was doing and he produced beautiful lettuces. He lived a healthy outdoor life and therefore it took me a long time to discover why his skin was in such a poor condition. Finally, I asked him to provide me with samples of all the fertilisers, herbicides, pesticides, etc. he used in his work. I then discovered that one additive, used for colouring, was clearly the offending factor. I put him on a desensitising programme, he stopped using the colouring, and his skin cleared up completely. This little tale reminds me of an elderly patient who checked some of the lettuces we produced in our organic kitchen garden. When I passed her she showed me a lettuce which contained a healthy slug and her comment was that if a slug could live on it, so could she. She was right, because some artificial additives such as chemical fertilisers and colourings are often used to make our food look more appetising, yet all too often they can be the cause of an allergic reaction. The skin will demonstrate the fact that inside the body there is a turmoil of objection because the body does not take kindly to such substances.

It goes without saying that a healthy diet and personal hygiene are very important for the skin. If we want to protect the skin, relaxation and sound sleep are also necessary. Everybody has had some spots or pimples at some time in their lives, but they ususally grow out of it. In constrast, a condition such as impetigo is often the sign of a streptococcus or staphylo-coccus bacterial infection, and such conditions should be treated immediately because they will spread rapidly. This is also true of a minor infection of the hair roots called folliculitis, or ringworm infection. If these conditions are allowed to get out of hand it will take more to overcome them. There are some very good natural antibiotics that can be used, for example Echinaforce, Phyto-Biotic and Seven Herb cream. These remedies, if taken in time, can help to overcome ringworm or folliculitis relatively quickly. The same goes for candida, or any fungal infection. The sooner it is treated the better, and remedies such as *Spilanthes* or *Harpagophytum* will help to rebalance the situation. Viral infections such as the common wart may be treated with the homoeopathic remedy *Thuja*.

What about herpes conditions, such as a cold sore, which is a herpes infection on the lip? How worried we are when we develop a cold sore, and yet it can be treated so quickly with a natural remedy such as Herpilyn. This is one of the finest remedies based on melissa extract, lemon balm and allantoin, and I have used it successfully in the treatment of many cold sores, scabs, fever blisters, etc.

A very uncomfortable condition, which is usually contracted in hot and damp conditions, such as in swimming pools and saunas, is symptomised by itching or a painful feeling on and around the anus. This is a nasty irritation that recurrently plagues the people it affects, and I can remember one gentleman in Australia admitting that it nearly made him suicidal. Two products that have helped quite a number of people to overcome this condition are Herpilyn and VyrBrit. I saw one poor lady recently who was not only suffering from shingles, but also had a herpes infection on her lower lip and on the anus. I prescribed *Avena sativa* (twice a day, fifteen drops) to help her nervous system, some Urticalcin and Viral Plex capsules, and VyrBrit to help the herpes condition. I also advised her to dab the skin affected by shingles alternately with a solution of Molkosan and the juice extracted from leeks. This treatment may be smelly, but it is highly effective, and with its help her condition soon improved.

Other skin diseases such as psoriasis, eczema and acne I have written about in detail in my book *Skin Diseases*, and here I intend to say no more than that it should always be remembered that diet plays a major role.

It is often claimed that the sun is a great healer for certain skin conditions. Certainly, natural sunshine is of great benefit, and the responsible use of artificial sunlight may also be helpful, but always use common sense. I am sad to say that I have seen many skin conditions, some of them leading to skin cancer, which were partially self-induced because no care was taken. In some cases it is better to avoid strong sunshine. For example, I had a young female patient who was an albino. She was most anxious to get some colour on her skin, but I had no option but to advise her to stay out of the sun altogether.

The pigment melanin is produced in the cells called melanocytes, and protects the sensitive part of all cells. However, we must be careful not to overdo sunbathing. We know that ultraviolet rays can be helpful, but please remember that they also can be detrimental, especially in excess. One of the biggest problems I have is with my multiple sclerosis patients, who love to lie in the sun but feel totally drained when they have done so, because it is not good for them. Protective creams or lotions will help to prevent the skin from burning or becoming too sensitive. The Sans Soucis range of protective creams is very helpful when sunbathing. When sunbathing is done sensibly, it may benefit conditions such as acne, psoriasis and eczema, as long as one keeps to the rules.

Over the years I have learned a great deal from treating people who suffer from skin problems such as burns, traumatic skin eruptions or scars. I am a great advocate of cosmetic acupuncture and homoeopuncture and, in many cases, this can be useful for scars, wrinkles and crow's feet. When such conditions can be dealt with satisfactorily, the emotional system gains in confidence. I have treated many people who have developed a complex about their skin problems, and I have usually been able to help with one or more of the therapies mentioned.

One of my best friends is a highly regarded plastic surgeon and we have often discussed the relief that he has been able to give people by removing certain offensive marks or features. The other day I saw a lady who had been badly burned in a house fire. She had severe scarring and my medical friend had managed to make a great improvement in her condition, but the scars were still clearly visible. However, with the help of cosmetic acupuncture and certain skin products, both she and I had reason to feel happy with our efforts. We may think that plastic surgery is something new, but let me tell you that over two thousand years ago in India, skin grafts and transplants were being undertaken, although it was naturally done in a more simple way. Nowadays, science has moved so far that much more can be done in this field.

If we need to help the skin, we can use sensible products to boost the immune system, such as Imuno-Strength, or a complex vitamin preparation such as Health Insurance Plus. These products will help the skin perform its tremendous function of maintaining a barrier against attacks from harmful foods and atmospherical influences. A healthy skin is also a useful barrier against bacterial and viral agents and therefore the diet is vitally important. This becomes clear when we look at the structure of the skin, which is dependent on keratin. This substance is found in the cells of the epidermis, where it helps to maintain the skin's texture and complexion and also fends off any bacteria that may be attacking the body.

The assimilation process of the skin is a necessary bodily function and I am not pleased when I hear that people use strong anti-perspirants. Many people have a complex about their smelly feet. They will use the strongest possible means to close off the sweat glands; but this is unwise. It is much better to solve this problem by sprinkling some borax in the shoes at night time. This does not stop the sweating, but it does neutralise the smell, and everybody should then be happy. From time to time take, twice a day, fifteen drops of Nephrosolid in a cup of Golden Grass Tea, as this is also helpful. Please be very wary of cheap deodorants because these sometimes contain aluminium. It is better to use a crystal preparation because any damage inflicted on that part of the skin can eventually lead to bigger problems.

These conditions are mentally, physically and emotionally influenced. Emotional tensions, fear or hormonal imbalances can cause excessive perspiration and medical advice may be necessary to keep this under control. Good circulation is important, as we have seen earlier in this book. Constipation, which often influences the circulation, also needs to be regulated. The hypothalamus works as a thermostat and the hormonal balance often needs a little help. Vitamins E and D are important, and it is surprising what can be achieved when the appropriate remedies are used.

Sometimes a stronger antibiotic is needed, as I saw with a patient whose skin was broken. The human body defends itself against invading microbes by a combination of pre-existing defence mechanisms and acquired immunity. In the front lines of defence are mechanical barriers such as the skin and epithelial cells, lining the air passages and the gastro-intestinal walls. The air passages, eyes and digestive system are protected by fluid secretions. Tears contain enzymes and wash away bacteria and ways, if not *the* best way, of using essential oils. Because our nasal passages have a direct line of contact with the brain, undiluted essential oils work almost immediately to relieve problems like sudden stress, depression, headaches, respiratory disorders and insomnia. Some of the oils which help in these conditions are listed below:

Sudden stress: basil, juniper, lavender, cedarwood, neroli, rose.
Depression: basil, bergamot, clary-sage, thyme, chamomile,
                 camphor, geranium, lavender, frankincense, jasmine,
                 neroli, patchouli, rose, sandalwood, ylang-ylang.
Headaches: lemon, eucalyptus, aniseed, chamomile, lavender.
Asthma: basil, cajuput, lemon, sage, thyme, aniseed, cypress,
                 hyssop, lavender, marjoram, melissa, peppermint, pine,
                 rosemary, savory, benzoin, clove, origanum.
Sinus problems: basil, eucalyptus, lemon, neroli, lavender,
                 peppermint, pine, clove.
Insomnia: basil, chamomile, camphor, juniper, lavender,
                 marjoram, neroli, rose, sandalwood, ylang-ylang.

Water is also a very useful carrier, especially when the oils are added to a warm bath. For all of the above complaints (except asthma, as the hot water makes the oils evaporate too quickly and they then become too powerful for an asthmatic to cope with), plus general aches and pains, poor circulation, ongoing stress, arthritis, menstruation problems and certain skin conditions, six to eight drops of the appropriate essential oils in the bath will produce amazing results in most cases.

Some oils that help these additional conditions are as follows:

Aches and pains: cajuput, coriander, caraway, eucalyptus, sage,
                     thyme, black pepper, chamomile, camphor,
                     juniper, lavender, marjoram, rosemary, clove,
                     ginger, nutmeg, origanum.
Poor circulation: lemon, black pepper, camphor, cypress, juniper,
                     rosemary, benzoin, rose, ginger.
Ongoing stress: basil, bergamot, clary-sage, petit-grain, thyme,
                     chamomile, geranium, juniper, lavender,
                     marjoram, melissa, benzoin, cedarwood, jasmine,
                     patchouli, rose, sandalwood.
Painful menstruation: cajuput, sage, aniseed, chamomile, cypress,
                     juniper, marjoram, melissa, peppermint, rosemary,

foreign objects. They also contain lysozymes which will kill bacteria. These should be considered the body's first line of defence.

If the skin is punctured or broken, free entry is allowed to bacteria and a complex set of reactions can trigger an acute inflammation. The damaged tissue is then amply supplied with phagocytes and white blood cells, sent by the bloodstream with proteins, to immobilise, neutralise and finally destroy the threatening invaders. In so doing the body has alerted its second line of defence. Those organisms that escape destruction through acute inflammation, trigger the alarm for more help. The body then produces specific antibodies that can bind themselves to hostile microbes and destroy them. It takes one to two weeks for the immune response to reach its peak the first time the body is challenged by a specific organism. After that, the body has a specific kind of memory that allows the alert response to enter into action much more rapidly when the same organism appears again. This is cellular memory and cellular intelligence in reaction, to support survival – the strongest instinct in the physical universe.

The most common agents of disease are bacteria and viruses, which behave very differently from each other. Scientists have also found that disease-inducing micro-organisms behave differently in the laboratory than they do in the human body. Even under the microscope many micro-organisms, such as the AIDS virus, change so rapidly that it is difficult to study them.

Viruses must reproduce inside a cell, but little is known about how bacteria elude the body's immune system. It is known that a strong immune system, a minimum of endotoxins, and a healthy diet (with adequate digestion, assimilation and elimination), are effective allies to support that mysterious cell recognition after the first attack of the mechanism that produces antibodies. Moreover, modern science has recognised the importance of the thymus gland in relation to immunity. The thymus gland, as mentioned in the section on the endocrine system, is of great importance here. Skin infections can be caused by the most common germs. The skin is the most important organ of the body with regard to elimination. Our body contains over two million sweat glands, and in order to have perfect health each sweat gland must be able to fulfil its particular task or activity. Through the pores of the skin, or sweat glands, we cast out the poisons that can harm the body. If the skin and glands are not active, there will be trouble in the blood, the kidneys and in the bowels. When these glands are active, they dispose of the detrimental acids from within the body. They also eliminate broken down minerals and tissues from our body.

There are two facts that are very noticeable and they will prove how necessary it is that these glands work in harmony with the rest of the body. First, when we perspire, the odour from the dead gases is still evident. Next, as proof of the elimination of dead tissue and decomposed minerals, you will find that when the sweat glands of the face become inactive, it is very visible inasmuch that blackheads develop. If you squeeze these from the outer ends of the glands, upon examination you will notice they are of a soft pasty substance. This is decomposed mineral and broken down tissue coming out through the pores. If elimination by way of the skin is not working properly, and has insufficient strength to cast out this mineral, but allows it to accumulate in the sweat gland and become a blackhead, then the process of elimination is blocked. The dead gases forming inside the body, which are supposed to be eliminated through the sweat glands, remain within. When they reach the skin and are unable to escape, they condense and turn into moisture, which settles in different parts of the body and causes the flesh, skin and organism to decay. This moisture has been termed 'old water', and weighs as much as 16 or 18 lb per gallon, while the specific gravity of fresh water is 8 lb per gallon.

Now for the sweat glands. When the glands fail to eliminate this refuse, it is taken into the lymphatic system and poured back into the red blood, and must be carried away through the bowels and kidneys, in which case the kidneys would have to eliminate sixteen times as much as they do normally. When this 'old water' begins to accumulate in the body, it makes the flesh become hard and bloated. This in turn interferes with the sweat glands.

Naturally there is less heat in the lower part of the body than there is in the head or chest, or the palms of the hands, and this is why many people perspire freely through the forehead, the palms of the hands and under the arms. Perspiration is more noticeable in the lower part of the body as there are many sweat glands that are kept open and free by the growing of hair from the inside of the skin out through the pores, which naturally give an outlet for perspiration. The odour from perspiration in this part of the body is as strong, if not stronger, than it is under the arms. The hair under the arms is supposed to keep the sweat glands free from blockage.

It is possible to locate any of the organs of the body that are out of order by paying attention to the skin. If the circulation is poor, a cold spot will appear over the heart. If the circulation is good, the entire chest will be warm. Lung or bronchial disorders may be detected by laying the hand on the upper part of the chest, directly under the collar bone. If the trouble is in the stomach or the duodenum, then the cold spot will appear on the front of the body below the diaphragm, just below the ribs. If the trouble is in the reproductive organs you will find a cold area just above the pelvic bone. The cold area in the case of ovarian problems appears nearer the hip bone. If the rectum is affected or there are piles, the cold spot will be found on the back over the sacrum. The indication of trouble in the kidneys will appear on the back just below the twelfth dorsal vertebra or the ribs.

Every organ in the body will thus indicate its condition by this symptom. When there is trouble in the eyes, ears and throat, you will find cold spots on the head, the back of the neck, the shoulders and arms, and above the location area of each organ of the body, for each organ of the body perspires as does the brow, and if for any reason the perspiration is checked, a cold spot develops. If the liver is not working properly there will be a cold spot over the liver as the action of the sweat glands will have stopped. As the perspiration leaves the body in other areas there will be a peculiar odour signifying retarded action in the liver. At times, the odour of the body may be like that of the stomach and bowels, or like that of the kidneys after an action.

It is possible to locate the cause of any problems by passing the palms of the hands over the flesh. When reaching a cold spot, it will become evident that the organ beneath needs attention. If the gall bladder is impaired, or the gall duct, a cold spot will be found on the right side of the body just at the bottom of the diaphragm near the bottom of the ribs. You may find a cold spot for the pancreas and the spleen on the opposite side of the body, at the left side just at the bottom of the ribs.

If the cause of distress is in the breathing or in the respiratory system, then right at the end of the breast bone is the centre for the solar plexus, which will take care of the breathing in a very short time. It must be understood that this is the greatest nerve centre – called a plexus – of the body which connects groups of nerves extending to all organs of the body, and treatment from this centre will immediately generate warmth from the minerals passing into the body, and into each and every organ.

The soles of the feet play a major role in the elimination process. Many people have developed serious problems affecting the kidneys and the lower limbs by trying to inhibit perspiration with the use of various solutions and medicines. The old remedy, if perspiration of the feet was excessive and offensive, was to bathe the feet in a solution made with a teaspoon of borax. This will relieve the odour, but it also has a detrimental effect because it seals the pores of the feet and inhibits perspiration. Large amounts of poison leave the body through the sweat glands in the feet, so this would be unwise. Many people have also ruined their health by applying solutions under the arms to check perspiration.

Walking, swimming and cycling, in fact any exercise taken in the fresh air is very good for the skin. Skincare products are plentiful, but we should be critical and ensure that the products we select are compatible with our skin. Many years ago I was asked to join the Committee of the Food and Drugs Association in Amsterdam. During the time I served on that committee we encountered some very strange complaints. Certain brands of cosmetics or perfumes caused skin problems, and some products were actually considered to be carcinogenic. An elderly doctor took the initiative to set up an alternative branch of this committee. Some of the natural products also failed the test, but fortunately there is much greater control nowadays. I remember that the skincare products I was most impressed with and were of the highest standard, were from a company called Sans Soucis. I was sufficiently interested to visit this company in the Black Forest in Germany and was surprised to learn that they trade in twenty-five countries all over the world. I have since then used some of their products in my clinics and my patients have been delighted with the results. Some of the most prescribed product lines are briefly described below:

Skin Repair Line with Repair Complex

This programme is designed for the treatment of skin that has diminished elasticity or pronounced wrinkles, caused by ultraviolet light; for skin suffering from harmful environmental influences; as a prophylactic measure against damage caused by ultraviolet light.

Sensitive Skin Line

A treatment programme designed for dry, sensitive skin with oil deficiency or with moisture deficiency, and for reddened or nervous skin.

Clear Skin Line

A series of products specifically devised for either oily or dry skin with impurities.

When I have treated a patient with cosmetic acupuncture for severe skin damage I may advise the use of a cover stick for any skin blemishes, and this has been most successful, especially in the early stages before the full benefits of the treatment become apparent.

I find that especially in Britain more people have a very sensitive skin, for which I may advise Echinaforce — twice a day, twenty drops before meals — and the remedy *Viola tricolor*. If we look at this flower, a three-leaved wild pansy, of a velvety texture, multi- and vibrantly coloured, it does not take too much imagination to see why this flower is meant to enhance the complexion. Depending on the patient, I may also recommend that they use Hair and Skin Capsules with some supplementary vitamin E.

For acne, especially among younger patients, I mostly start by prescribing Echinaforce, and an excellent product in these circumstances is Acne-Zyme, sometimes taken in combination with *Viola tricolor*.

A healthy skin depends to a large extent on a healthy body and all the advice I have provided above will help the skin to show beauty within and without.

21

Healthy Hair

A healthy head of hair is like a crown on the body. It is often said that hair makes a woman. Hair loss or baldness is more common among men, but women are no less disturbed when faced with these problems. It is often seen that emotional trauma affects hair growth, or it can even turn the hair white prematurely, as in the case of Queen Marie Antoinette, whose hair supposedly turned white overnight during the French Revolution. Certainly, the hair will express the problems of the soul.

People often complain about the condition of their hair. Whether it is greasy, dry, or unmanageable, hair problems are probably linked to the individual's general health. The best advice for women with greasy hair is to let it grow. The skin of the scalp is covered with countless follicles from which hair will naturally grow to its own length, and enough oils are secreted to keep the hair in perfect condition. When the hair is cut very short, these follicles still produce the natural amount of oil, which makes the hair appear greasy.

When women dye their hair, it may become too dry. Essential fatty acids as found in Evening Primrose oil may help to restore the balance in the production of natural oils. In olden days it was said that the seat of the soul is the symbol of strength and power in man. Animals are protected against the loss of body heat by their hair growth or pelt, but for man this is no longer required. The scalp has between 100,000 and 200,000 hairs. As this hair grows from the follicle of the upper skin, each hair is also determined from birth. No wonder that the Creator of man said that even the hairs on one's head are counted.

Keratin helps our hair to grow roughly one-third of a millimetre each day. Special cells conduct the colouring of each hair, although hair colour is decided genetically. It is wonderful to know that hair grows all the time in its own follicle. Each hair is replaced after three years and it is said that 40–100 hairs can fall out every day and are replaced by slowly growing new ones. Hair loss, or total baldness, have historically been of great interest, and although there are many factors that determine hair growth the hormonal system plays a particularly significant role, so once again it becomes clear that the condition of the hair is greatly influenced by the harmony between the three bodies of man.

Hormone treatment can cause loss of hair or stimulate the growth of hair. This reaction is genetically decided and spontaneous hair loss can also be caused by a variety of factors, usually influenced by atmospherical imbalance. Hair loss at the front is usually caused by a hormonal imbalance, while hair loss at the back is determined by genetic influences. Hair loss in patches is usually caused by an infection. Sometimes people with excessive hair loss are worried that they may be bald for life, but this is not always the case. Women in particular can get very upset about hair loss and they immediately feel they are no longer attractive. For both men and women a good head of hair is important.

I remember a teacher who had lost most of her hair because of shock. She had to wear a wig, and when the children found out, she was understandably embarrassed when teased about it. Once or twice one of the older boys had even pulled off her wig. She begged me for help to restore her hair growth as quickly as possible, and once we started with some natural remedies and a new dietary programme her hair began to grow back again. Initially, this regrowth can lack colour, but gradually the normal hair colour usually returns. She was delighted with the outcome of a liver-cleansing remedy, Boldocynara together with Priorin, and a hair-growth promoting capsule called Healthy Hair.

The shaft of a human hair consists of a special protein called keratin, of which the amino acid L-cysteine is a component. Vitamins C and E are included in the Healthy Hair formula because of their roles in the general health and well-being of the capillaries, which supply the hair follicles with nutrients. It also includes a series of B vitamins at the appropriate levels.

It is important to have any split ends trimmed regularly and to use a good shampoo and hair lotions such as onion or nettle lotion, which give the hair a boost. I remember a young girl who, because of a slight hormonal dysfunction, lost all her hair. She became desperate and understandably sensitive about this. She was studying German at the time and because of that I quoted an expression made famous by Schiller, a German scientist: *Es ist der Geist der sich den Körper baut*. (It is the spirit that builds the body.) This confirms that the emotional body is very much involved in our physical well-being. If a woman loses her hair it is more complicated than in the case of a man, as women have one extra chromosome compared to men. This girl was given several remedies, including wheatgerm oil capsules, Evening Primrose oil, and Maxi-Hair, and slowly her hair growth returned. When I see her now, I can tell it has not done her any harm because the newly-grown hair is of beautiful quality. Emotional trauma has often been the cause of hair loss, and I have certainly been told some interesting stories by my patients.

Sometimes, after a shock the face may turn white, and when we are worried or frightened this may have an immediate effect on the digestive system, or on the bowels, possibly causing diarrhoea. This frequently happens to people who suffer from examination fear. People who are frightened of losing their hair, are more likely to actually lose it, because of their negative attitude and worrying. Strength of mind is so important and a good example of this can be seen when trying to get rid of warts. If some considerate or superstitious adult volunteers to 'buy' a wart from a child, and promises that child that within fourteen days he or she will take over that wart, then often that wart will have disappeared within that time span. Another old wife's tale was to cover the wart with some fresh meat, bury the piece of meat in the ground, and by the time that the piece of meat had rotted away, the wart would be gone. It was a well-known treatment in its day, and it worked because the mind is stronger than the body.

With different kinds of hair loss like ariatra or alopecia totalis, it is essential to have a positive mind, or else there is no hope that the hair will ever return. Some people are so obsessed with the threat of hair loss, that because of the worry they will lose it. Julius Caesar promised his hairdresser half of Rome if he could make his hair return. It is sad how many people with hair loss problems are taken in by glib advertising, often lacking any scientific basis, but where the products are a good money-spinner for the manufacturers, who prey on people's vulnerability.

When dandruff occurs something should be done as quickly as possible. Massage the scalp regularly so that the skin covering the scalp is kept supple. In some cases it is wise to take a protein deficiency formula, which will also help the hormonal system and produce more adrenalin and thyrosine, which creates more melanin. It is essential to eat plenty of fruit and vegetables, because this also plays a major role in hair growth.

Massaging the scalp and brushing with a hairbrush which is not too hard are very important. I find that with all hair conditions it is helpful to take, twice a day, five tablets of Urticalcin, together with the herbal extract *Galeopsis*, and if a woman has problems with her ovaries, as is often the case, the homoeopathic remedy *Ovarium 3X*. Dandruff often indicates a lack of vitamin A, and this may need to be supplemented, but only if the patient is sure that she is not pregnant. Diluted Molkosan can be used in the last rinse after the hair has been washed. This is also helpful if the scalp is itchy. Sometimes I use acupuncture or the old-fashioned high-frequency apparatus to stimulate the hair root back to life. The hair root is often lacking in keratin and stimulation helps to keep this production going. Following a healthy diet containing fruit, vegetables and brown rice, together with the remedies Urticalcin, Boldocynara and Maxi-Hair, will speed up the results. However, if the results are very slow I may also introduce the Hair and Skin Nutrition preparation, which provides a balanced combination of vitamins, minerals and other natural factors to nutritionally support the many systems involving and maintaining healthy hair.

Essential fatty acids (EFAs) play an important role in the body's natural oils that keep the scalp in good condition. Sometimes EFAs are known as vitamin F, and combined with a vitamin B complex preparation, they can help to maintain a healthy head of hair. The crown of the head, in a healthy growth of hair, often reflects what is happening inside the body. Outwardly, we can quickly see what is happening internally. Often it is simple to rectify problems of hair growth, dandruff and greasy or dry hair. If need be you may call on the help of a good practitioner so that this attractive part of the body is kept as healthy as possible.

22

Healthy Feet

Some time ago Dr Vogel and I were walking in the mountains when he suddenly said to me: 'The feet – they are important to health.' As we were in the midst of discussing a serious subject, I was astonished when he suddenly came out with this unexpected reaction and the conversation turned to the subject of feet. It goes without saying that the feet are important, because they carry the weight of the entire body. Dr Vogel, who is by now in his nineties, is still able to walk in the beautiful surroundings of his house, and that in itself proves that he has taken good care of his feet. He also believes in barefoot therapy and still walks with bare feet as often as he can. This, of course, is another important matter, because by using the bare feet, all the reflex points and acupuncture points in the feet are being used and stimulated – and walking barefoot on gravel is particularly beneficial. A barefooted walk in the snow is excellent for the circulation. Today, we have grown away from such methods, and I wonder if it is because they appear too simple and therefore not scientifically acceptable. Barefoot sole therapy is still widely practised in the East, with excellent results.

If we consider what our feet do for us they certainly deserve more consideration than they are generally given. In ancient times, the Egyptians developed reflexology, and it is sad that for so long this treatment method was forgotten. However, we must be grateful that reflexology is now enjoying a revival. Recently, I met some therapists who have developed a method of stimulating some of the pressure points on the feet for slimming purposes, which are supposed to burn up fats more quickly. These specific pressure points relate to the endocrine system, and in a later chapter on the metabolism I will come back to this.

Reflexology is based on the principle of a large number of zones in the feet, each relating to specific organs. There are zones for the heart, liver, kidneys and endocrine glands. There are also zones to speed up the metabolism – and these happen to lie in the ear. Like the feet, the ears contain a great number of pressure points and zones.

It is easy to neglect the feet, but just think how often we remark or notice that our feet are tired. Many people have a great deal of hard skin on their feet, and we have all experienced occasions when we have wanted to kick off our shoes because our feet were burning. Of a long list of foot problems just think about how many you have experienced: hard skin, sweaty feet, corns, blisters, ingrowing toenails, athlete's foot, fungi, chilblains, calcium deposits, gout, bunions or verrucas. It really can be quite a daunting list. When our feet serve us faithfully, we tend to forget about them, but if one of the above conditions plagues us, then we suddenly realise the need for healthy feet. Then we suddenly look for help. At the end of the day most people are happy to kick off their shoes. That usually means that we have not taken sufficient care, i.e. the shoes we have been wearing may have been too tight, or the socks or stockings may be too tight or of the wrong material, restricting the circulation. We rarely consider the fact that our feet should be accorded the same care that we give to our teeth. We think it is perfectly normal to brush our teeth twice a day, while many people will admit that they do not wash their feet even once a day. Diabetics should take particular care of their feet, because when the blood circulation slows they will experience less feeling, and they are therefore advised to exercise the feet, for example by walking or swimming, taking care not to get blisters or cuts.

Foot-baths can be very therapeutic for a number of medical conditions, such as congestion, head colds or insomnia, and they are of great benefit as a circulatory stimulant. If you really want to give the feet a treat, you will require two large containers, large enough to soak the feet in and allow the water to reach well up the calf. One of these containers should be filled with comfortably hot water, with some more hot water kept close at hand to top up the water in the container in order to keep the temperature at a comfortable level. The second container should contain cold water. Immerse both feet in the hot water for two or three minutes. Then move the feet to the container with the cold water, keeping them there for some thirty seconds. Meanwhile, add some more hot water to the first container and place the feet in there again. Continue the alternate foot-bath treatment for a period of up to half an hour. This treatment is a powerful circulatory stimulant and can be used in cases of poor circulation.

Yet another simple foot exercise is what is called 'the cold dip', and this is a treatment method I learned some years ago in India. This exercise has to be done each morning before getting out of bed and each night before retiring. Place a basin of cold water by the bed with a towel at the side. On waking up in the morning, place both feet into the water. Having counted to ten, remove the feet onto the towel to damp dry them. Exercise the toes as if trying to pick up a marble. Repeat this between ten and thirty times. On retiring, follow the same procedure as in the morning. You will find your feet will be as warm as toast when you go to bed. To obtain the full benefits, this exercise should be done for a minimum of sixty days.

To treat a verruca, athlete's foot, or another fungal condition, Molkosan should be used. This remedy is ideally suited for these conditions and it should be dabbed onto the relevant area twice a day. Seven Herb Cream is excellent for all-over foot care, as is St John's wort oil. A fungal condition, or calcium deposits, especially under the nails, can be greatly relieved by a remedy called Propolis Wart Tincture, and this is also very helpful for persistent warts. For brittle nails, whether on the fingers or toes, take five tablets of Urticalcin twice a day, and as this complaint is fairly common, it may sometimes be necessary to use a slightly stronger remedy such as Hair and Skin Capsules, which are also very good. For circulatory problems affecting the extremities, Hyperisan, Urticalcin and a vitamin E supplement should be taken.

Most people with varicose veins or haemorrhoids also experience cold feet. This is the reason that great therapists like Rolf always devoted an entire treatment to manipulating the feet, generally upon the second visit. In persistent cases she would pay attention to the feet during successive visits as well. Under no circumstances would the feet be overlooked. The soles of the feet contain more nerves than any other exposed area of the body, with the exception of the anal region.

It has been claimed that nerve pressure on the feet can be communicated via the tibial and sciatic nerves to the solar plexus, thus affecting the sympathetic system. Frequently, the feet will be so tense that the bones are almost consolidated. There should be movement between each of the main bones, and when the foot is relatively free a twisting type of manipulation can readily induce this movement, and in most cases this is an audible release that can be felt and heard. Many times with rheumatic or arthritic patients I have noticed that they are flat-footed, and I have lost count of the times that I have had to adjust the cuboid bones in the feet. Whenever I see a patient with a 'Charlie Chaplin' posture I immediately know that I will have to treat the feet, which are an immediate indication of other problems.

The relationship between pain and magnetic distortion is direct and unfailing. It can be stated as a physiological law and I have often wondered why Kirlian made his diagnosis using the feet and hands, on the physical, mental and the emotional bodies. I am sure that the endocrine system plays a great role. In the feet as well as in the hands all the reflexes of the endocrines are present and therefore reflexology can bring great relief when the practitioner uses the right hand on the correct places, standing on the correct side of the patient, so that negative and positive are in balance and in tune with the south and north poles. There exists some informative literature on the feet by well-known authors such as Fitzgerald, Bressler, Reilly, Daglish and Lust, and more recently by Eunice Ingham, author of the excellent book *Stories that the Feet Can Tell*. For many years these foot reflex methods only seemed to achieve partial success. It was later, when I had looked further into body zones and the importance of the occiput, that a greater degree of success with patients was obtained, and after fewer treatments.

Dr Leonard Allan always made it very clear that the head is the positive pole, while the feet are the negative pole. The hands are neutral. I will remind you again of the analogy with the battery of a car, where right is positive and left is negative. Right is always looking for negative, but in the middle is the neutral zone. The hands in this case act as the neutral zone. It is only when the entire body is balanced that success may be achieved.

Centuries ago, the Chinese and the Indonesians used the feet to diagnose and treat illness. This was their method of exciting the reflexes, short of awakening the responses. Acupuncture is a reflex therapy and acts on the autonomic system. Although some acupuncturists disagree on this point, this is a fact and a law. The sooner they accept the fact of reflex action, the sooner their labour will be rewarded.

Problems such as bunions, callouses, and hammer toes tell us that there are inherent distortions in the body. Every part of the body is in touch with the world around us and these experiences are reflected through the body and the mind. All matter settles at the lowest point, in this instance the feet or the negative pole. We will find all the hormonal reflexes there, so the three bodies of man are also tangible in the feet.

The science of endocrinology embraces the internal secretions of all the ductless glands and this is something to which we ought to pay much more attention. The secretions from these glands are discharged directly into the bloodstream and are very potent and necessary to the body for its daily use. The ductless glands are the supply depot for the living organisms. The nutrition from our food – indeed, our entire physical life – is regulated by these all-important glands or centres, even to the kind of skin, the colour of hair, and the strength of muscles. Many of the glands that have ducts and form an external secretion also form an internal secretion, such as the liver, the pancreas, the membranes of the stomach and the intestines. The endocrine glands show how much they need our help and it is here where reflexology and aromatherapy can be used so advantageously. It is encouraging to know how many contact points there are in the human body, especially on the feet and the head. We can use essential oils and aromatherapy oils or essences to help to relieve a number of conditions. A well-trained aromatherapist or reflexologist can achieve wonders with either the feet or the head. A cranial osteopath will have been taught which points to use and many of these have been mentioned in my book *Body Energy* together with guidelines on their use for specific circumstances.

This was again confirmed a few months ago during a radio interview. The telephone lines were open for questions, and a lady caller spoke to me about her husband who had remained unconscious for weeks following a traffic accident. The coma was so severe that he had not yet shown any sign of regaining consciousness. I told this caller at which point on the cranium she should rub some St John's wort oil with her thumb. She followed my advice and even as she was doing so he regained consciousness. She excitedly phoned again during a consecutive programme and I told her that she had been only a mechanism, because it was her husband's body itself that had done what was necessary.

Having related the above experience, I am reminded of another friend from the broadcasting world. She is a very attractive young woman, but I had always noticed when in conversation with her, that she was very tense. I often spoke with her, but I felt that there was very little feedback and therefore she had to learn to relax. I recommended acupuncture treatment, and I also advised her on certain reflexology practices, using some of my own oils. On a subsequent visit to the broadcasting studio, this young friend walked in and I knew immediately that she was very keyed up and totally frustrated. I decided to have a word with her and she agreed to undergo treatment. I selected certain pressure points on the feet and ankles, and some on the head, and I used some of these oils. I then purposely left her alone and returned some ten minutes later. I found her sobbing, and gave her some Emergency Essence to help her to calm down. Then we talked, and this time she opened up and poured out her heart. This was a perfect example of complete disharmony between the three bodies of man. Now she is a changed person and anyone who has observed her will realise that. I am sure that in future she will become one of our leading broadcasters, because the full capabilities of this young lady, although excellent, had remained hidden by emotional trauma she had not previously faced up to. Although she disliked me for bringing her problem to the surface and showing this flaw in her character, she realised that it had been a blessing, and will be decisive in her future.

All natural therapies aim to keep the body in balance, naturally endeavouring to bring harmony between all the different physical body systems – and the mind. When you correct an imbalance, good health will prevail.

Most people seem to want others to take the responsibility for their health, when in fact the balance is restored much more quickly when patients take an active and positive part in bringing about their own recovery, both physically and mentally.

Actually, prime responsibility must always lie with the patient, assisted with expert guidance from the therapist. As far as aromatherapy treatments are concerned, it is advisable for therapists to give the client 'homework' in one or both of the following forms:

- pure oils to inhale and/or put in the bath
- mixed oils or lotions to apply to the face and/or body, not only to help the cause of the problem, but also to alleviate the symptoms that are upsetting to the patient.

The body has its own natural inbuilt ability to heal itself and when it does need help, natural therapies together with a positive approach on the part of both therapist and patient can usually do the job without resorting to synthetic pills and tablets with their often detrimental side-effects.

An interesting test was recently conducted in the field of conventional medicine. A number of people with the same health problem was divided into two groups. One group saw a consultant who gave them positive encouragement, showing a real interest in their problems and giving them a positive diagnosis and an optimistic forecast. The consultant for the second group followed a more negative and disinterested approach. I need not tell you that a much higher rate of recovery was evident among the people in the first group.

During consultations (and this is the case for all complementary therapists with whom I have come into contact), it always pays to get the patient actively involved. Aromatherapists, unless they also have other specialised training, are not usually qualified to make a diagnosis. Fully trained personnel use the reflexes of the feet and ask pertinent questions to discover both the physical and mental state of the patient and, of course, they spend time listening, so that the emotional state of the whole person can be asssessed. From the answers they are given, it is possible to deduce which oils will be most likely to revitalise the systems of the body which are out of balance.

Aromatherapy involves using the aromas of essential oils to therapeutically revitalise and strengthen the cellular tissues. It should be stressed that I am talking of *essential oils* here, as nowadays a few people trade in 'aromatherapy oils', which are not necessarily the same as pure, unadulterated esssential oils. Apart from expressed volatile oils, all of which are found in the skins of citrus fruits, essential oils can be found in the petals, leaves, seeds, stems, bark or roots of various plants, bushes or trees, they are present in minute amounts, locked in tiny oil 'glands', which burst during distillation to release their precious oils.

When the entire plant is used, the concentration of healing power is necessarily spread over a greater area, so more plant material is needed to effect a similar result. Also, plants hold other healing properties in their structure, which are made use of in herbal medicine. Aromatherapists use only the esssential oils, which have quite a few advantages:

- They take up less space, so are much more convenient for travelling and holidays.
- They are ready for instant use, and will keep more or less indefinitely. The therapeutic qualities of some whole plants can change drastically after being stored for some time.
- The therapeutic effect is considerably magnified in the esssential oil as opposed to the whole plant.
- They can be used in a greater variety of ways.

It is important to know that some plants contain more essential oil than others, so therefore the cost can vary immensely. It is also important to know that a true essential oil, without adulteration of any kind, is of necessity more expensive than an oil of the same name which has been 'standardised', i.e. given a British Pharmaceutical standard. This may even mean that alterations have been made to the natural oil to enable it to conform with what may be a lower standard than many plants are capable of producing.

The highly concentrated nature of essential oils means that in order to use them for aromatherapy they must first be mixed with a 'carrier'. A prime example of such a carrier is air, which carries essential oils into our noses when we inhale from a tissue. In fact, inhalation is one of the best

	jasmine, tarragon.
PMT:	lavender, melissa, neroli, rose, geranium, chamomile, clary-sage.
Eczema:	sage, chamomile, hyssop, geranium, lavender, bergamot, juniper, sandalwood.
Sore throat:	eucalyptus, thyme, cajuput, cedarwood, sandalwood, lemon, tea tree.

Another way of using essential oils with water as the carrier is, I think, an excellent one. It is possible to make tea using essential oils. If possible, tannin-free teabags should be used, though ordinary ones will do to make a very weak basic brew. If you have a stomach upset you may choose to add two drops of peppermint and one drop of fennel to a teabag, over which you pour one and a half pints of nearly boiling water. Stir well and remove the teabag. Then drink one cup of tea three times a day, saving the rest in a jug in the fridge until it is needed again. It is great fun to experiment with teas to help you sleep, teas to relieve stress, teas for reviving the brain (if you have a lot of work to do), and all from one packet of tea and a few little bottles.

One of the most popular methods of using essential oils is by application to the skin. Professional aromatherapists use a vegetable oil as a carrier so that they can carry out the special massage techniques now associated with aromatherapy. Shiatsu pressures, lymphatic drainage and neuro-muscular massage, together with effleurage movements contribute to this form of massage, and it is one of the best and most pleasurable treatments that exist for dealing with stress and its associated problems.

A well-trained aromatherapist will mix a bottle of oils that have been used in your treatment for your own use at home. You may be given them in their pure form for inhalation, baths or teas, and also perhaps in a carrier oil or non-greasy lotion (the latter is much more pleasant to apply) for use after your bath or shower.

The skin responds well to the application of esssential oils in carrier oils, lotions or creams. A good quality aromatherapy skin-care range will rejuvenate the skin when used regularly, softening and smoothing its texture. People with problem skins, blocked sinuses, eczema or headaches, for example, can, with a specially formulated aromatherapy moisturising cream, take care of their skin at the same time as treating these problems. A hand lotion especially developed for arthritis patients, softens the skin while at the same time relieving the pain and making movement easier.

Our feet are our true servants and need all our attention. In their service they will tell us when something is wrong. Little alarm bells ring, such as cold feet, indicating circulation problems that could eventually develop into varicose veins or haemorrhoids, or even into chilblains. These conditions can also be helped and not only with reflexology, aromatherapy and essential oils: one can start using a simple foot-bath with a hot potato decoction or an oak bark decoction, together with Hyperisan, *Aesculus hippocastanum*, Urticalcin, or special homoeopathic remedies. Perspiration of the feet is often necessary, and people cause themselves lots of problems when they try to prevent it. Remember that it is nature freeing the body of fluid which usually contains waste material, and must not be stopped. If the smell is unpleasant, sprinkle some borax in the shoes, or try using some of the appropriate essential oils on the feet.

Take care of your feet and select your footwear carefully. If possible, try barefoot treatment or with some of the different hydrotherapy treatments, and your feet will serve you well.

23

Healthy Food

On one of my lecture tours in the United States I was invited to take part in a television broadcast on stress, menopausal and menstrual problems. I had not been prepared for the fact that I was to be joined by two ladies on the panel who were representatives from the food industry. It was whispered that apparently they were going to dispute some of the facts I had included in my book *Nature's Gift of Food*. When I met these ladies before the programme, they were very argumentative and hostile, and flatly stated that so-called health foods had nothing whatsoever to do with health. When we entered the studio I noticed an impressive display of junk food staring me in the face. When the interviewers asked a tall, skinny lady which was her favourite, she pointed to a large bottle of coloured, fizzy drink. She stated that she would drink two to three bottles of this a day, and in a challenging manner she added that she felt absolutely great. I had studied her before we went on the programme and now I asked her why she was ill. She vehemently denied that she was ill, but I told her that she was hyperactive and highly-strung, her hair was lifeless and her skin looked pasty. Mentally, physically and emotionally, all the evidence of her dietary indulgence was there. She was unable to deny that her appearance showed up all the shortcomings of her diet.

The other lady was a pleasant, considerably overweight person, and when she was asked about her favourite item from the display, she picked up a cake that looked like a cream doughnut, which I have been told is called locally a 'Susie Que'. She told us that a Susie Que was her favourite breakfast. I then asked her why she was ill, and she also denied it. I told her that she was suffering from allergy problems and had chronic sinusitis, and I also asked if her obesity was causing her any problems. She said no more but indicated with a little nod that I was right. That afternoon she came to see me as a patient.

In essence, what I want to look at in this chapter is the ways in which food can influence the three bodies of man, and the external evidence of incorrect nutrition. In the case of these two ladies I only had to look at them to discover that they had nutritional problems. The expression 'The danger is on your plate' holds a great deal of truth. It does not take long to discover that a child who eats too much sugar can become hyperactive. Nor does it take me long, when I visit female prisoners, and hear about their diets, to realise why they have emotional problems. I recognise the facts on prison visits, and I can clearly see why nutrition and the mind are so closely interrelated. Nor does it need a great deal of research to see why today there are so many cases of paratyphoid, food poisoning or an over-abundance of food – which spell out trouble for the mind, body and soul. I say this, even though I realise that many of my readers will respond to this with a measure of reservation.

However, if the soul or spirit of man is determined, it can overcome many controversial or detrimental situations – even famine or gross malnutrition. We only have to think of the pictures that were published at the end of the Second World War of the survivors of the concentration camps. It is not the case that these survivors were the strongest among those who originally entered these camps; it was more likely to be the strongest in spirit who managed to survive. I remember that even as a youngster I was puzzled by my father's return after the war, feeling grateful that he had survived. He had something in his life that was worth living for, and he held on to this to the bitter end. This was what carried him through that dreadful experience. When we look at people who have endured similar situations throughout the world, we can see that it is mostly a strong spirit that keeps them alive.

Mentally, the human brain does not give away the secrets of its mind. Emotionally, man does not tend to reveal what goes on inside. One certainty is that if there is emotional and mental balance, man will be physically much stronger than we can ever imagine.

I have read with great interest some press information on a study called *Personality and Individual Differences*, which is a report on a trial held among US school children. This was conducted by the Dietary Research Foundation, which was created as an independent charity in 1989 to conduct research into the effects of nutrition on human health and behaviour and, in particular, to investigate whether giving nutritional supplements to school children can improve their IQ. The Scientific Directorate comprised specialists in the field of nutrition, psychology, biostatistics, sociology and criminal justice. The extensive research programme, which was conducted among 615 school children aged 12–13 and 15–16 years, found that the average non-verbal IQ score of the group taking a formulation designed by the Dietary Research Foundation showed a significant improvement when compared with a group taking a placebo. This improvement was equivalent to more than four IQ points, moving an IQ score from a halfway point in the IQ league to a position where it was ahead of 62 per cent of the others. The likelihood of such a change occurring by chance is minimal. Improvements in individual IQ scores were independent of age, sex, school or starting IQ scores of the children.

Participants in the research programme were given two tablets daily, representing one of three different potencies of multivitamin and mineral tablets, or placebo tablets containing no active ingredients. The supplements contained all the vitamin and mineral elements known or thought to be essential nutrients (thirteen vitamins and ten minerals) and were taken for a full school term.

The conclusion was that supplementation with a particular range and strength of vitamins and minerals led to an improvement in average IQ score and this had occurred in children who would normally be considered as receiving sufficient nutrients in the diet.

Playfair is a suitable supplement, as it was specifically designed for children. This supplement is a combination of vitamins and minerals designed to overcome deficiencies and to help with concentration. Children who have problems with forthcoming examinations or general concentration can be helped by taking a a zinc supplement or *Ginkgo biloba*.

All over the world people seem to want to investigate nutrition. In 1992, for the first time in the UK, a White Paper was published on the *Health of the Nation*. This White Paper set out to promote public health across the whole community. During the last century many diseases have been controlled or eliminated, and now we have much better health as a result. This progress has not only added years to our lives, but also life to our years.

Many years ago I joined Dr Vogel at a lecture in Amsterdam in which he stressed that it is not the quantity of food but its quality that is important. The quantity is only of secondary importance, as long as the quality of the food intake is good. He also pointed out the importance of digesting our food properly, because this aids absorption. Absorption is even more important than food quality, because if assimilation or absorption is poor, this good-quality nutrition will make little or no difference to our health. It is a tremendous challenge laid down by the government in *Health of the Nation*, and everybody has a part to play. The government can provide advice, but ultimately the responsibility for our health lies with each and every single one of us. Therefore education is necessary and this becomes very clear to me in my public lectures when I see how many people are hungry for nutritional knowledge.

When I look at the general nutritional guidelines I am happy with what has been established so far, but we cannot stand still, because this is a fast-developing area. The *Sunday Times* of 16 October 1994 featured an interesting article entitled 'Eat up your Greens'. It is true that greens, or vegetables, are very important to the diet. This article claimed that water plants have been recognised by scientists as being the most nutritious, and that certain species of seaweed are now enjoying unprecedented popularity as food supplements. Not only will the blue-green algae boost vitality, but it will improve sleep, reduce allergies, stop migraines, reduce stress, alleviate PMT and boost the body's immune system. In that article it was even claimed to be a total food, so there is no need to worry about additional supplements.

Every day we learn about foods that will help to keep us healthy. Lately we have been able to read about the great benefits of an extract from grapefruit seeds, which can work as a natural antibiotic and help in the treatment of problems such as candida, bacteria and parasites. We often forget that many seeds have a nutritional value; for example, grape seeds are helpful in controlling cholesterol levels and pumpkin seeds benefit the urinary system.

It is common knowledge that the excessive consumption of refined sugar leads to dental caries. If the teeth – the hardest tissue in the oral cavity, which forms the first part of the digestive tract – are so easily affected and decayed by this highly concentrated carbohydrate, the question arises of what is it doing to the intestines. Damaging evidence has emerged from research conducted on the reflexes of the body as a whole of severe disturbance caused further down the digestive tract, and in the first part of the lower gut.

During the Second World War an eighteen-month study was carried out among tens of thousands of troops who were based in Russia. One of the conclusions of the medical officer who conducted the research was that sugar affected the gut and often caused peptic ulcers. Problems of anxiety, fatigue and deficiencies were noted amongst the troops. Sugar not only attacks the teeth, but also affects the levels of vitamins, minerals and trace elements in the body. It was McCarisson who stated that deficiencies in certain vitamins and minerals will lead to haemorrhages in various parts of the body, swelling of joints, skin imperfections, unhealthy gums, congestion of the bladder, gastro-intestinal disorders and stress.

In an earlier chapter I stated that the three main enemies of man are salt, sugar and stress. There is always a connection with the physical, mental and emotional bodies, and I have seen for myself that nutrition influences the brain, especially in the case of children. This link has also been confirmed by the studies I have undertaken with prisoners.

A female patient told me that twenty years ago, her hands would sometimes rise up in the air involuntarily, and she did not know why it was happening. A psychiatrist explained that half of her brain was asleep, while the other half was wide awake. The problem had started with strange sensations and she tried to get help, but nobody found out what was wrong. She told me that she even went to a clairvoyant, but it appeared that the problem was within herself and she was unable to control it. After a while, a homoeopathic practitioner did some allergy tests, and discovered that she was allergic to sugar, which affected her so much emotionally that she could not cope with life. Her life completely changed when she cut out sugar from her diet. I have seen this often, especially with hyperactive children who can be a great worry to their parents and teachers, but whose attitude changes when white sugar is banned from the diet. If we have to have sugar, it should be in the form of honey, unrefined soft brown sugar or demerara sugar.

Today, we have an abundance of so-called 'twentieth-century diseases', many of which are directly related to allergic reactions to specific foods that upset any one of the three bodies of man. This prevents harmony within the body. One of the latest, but fastest-growing, allergies is an adverse reaction to wheat. A whole range of artificial and chemical means are employed today in the production of wheat, and few people are aware of the fact that these additives can affect the brain. Many problems occur because of the highly increased number of chromosomes in the wheat grain, which is the reason why many people's bodies can no longer cope with this food. One of the signs that the body cannot cope is an unidentifiable skin disease. Wheat grains also contain more gluten than in the past, and this can affect certain parts of the body, and is thought to be contributory to serious conditions such as multiple sclerosis. During the Second World War in the Netherlands there were hardly any stomach problems, and I often wonder if this was because of the very low gluten intake. Sometimes when I detect a wheat allergy there is very little to differentiate between infections and disease. We can call it what we like, but disease is *dis-ease*, and with all disease there is a breakdown of cell tissue. If we call it life, we can say that cell tissue renewal is the physical process of life. Therefore it is necessary for any interference, even food which can interfere with this life process, to be avoided. Life is cell renewal, and this process cannot continue if sustained with only tinned fruit or a tin of tomato soup. Foods that are wholesome and nutritious are needed for this purpose and, holistically, the entire body will benefit. Degeneration and disease are two entirely separate processes: the first being autonomous breakdown of the metabolic function of building healthy replacement cell tissue – a nutritional problem – and the second being a breakdown of tissue because of attack by germs, viruses or allergies. Either of these will become a medical problem.

Often, a vitamin, mineral or trace element deficiency, or an allergy will provide the key, and sometimes a specific diet may help. Gluten, if taken in large quantities, is often the cause of stomach and bowel problems. This is very clearly the case in coeliac disease, but gluten sensitivity is often the key to other problems as well. In countries where gluten intake is low, the incidence of degenerative disease is also low.

I have designed a diet as part of the treatment for schizophrenia, which is a condition involving both mind and body. It becomes easier for a schizophrenic to regain balance when sugar and wheat are eliminated from the diet. It sometimes requires only a small dietary change to make a big impact. If we lived closer to nature we would know instinctively what was good for us to eat . A small bird, with a brain smaller than the size of a pea, will not eat a poisonous berry, while a child with a brain the size of a turnip will eat these greedily, and will then have to suffer the consequences. We have lost the instinctive knowledge required to differentiate between what is beneficial and what is harmful. We have to re-educate ourselves to choose according to our instincts, and by sharpening our instincts we will be investing in a happy future. If I was to take a plate full of gold pieces and some fruits and nuts and hold it in front of an animal, the instinct of the animal would be to go for the fruits and nuts. Man would immediately go for the gold, yet the correct diet and healthy food will be a golden investment for his own future, making his life richer, happier and healthier.

I once attended a lecture given by a professor of nutrition, which left a lasting impression on me. Some people considered her statements to be somewhat extreme, and they may have been right. She had a very attentive audience when she told them that a plant feeds on minerals, animals eat plants, man eats animals, but who feeds on man? It is sad to think that man, whose staple food is fruits and vegetables, also eats so many things that are not good for him. This scientist, in her talk, claimed that the answer to the question was that angels and fellow men feed on man. This statement is too extreme for my liking, but nevertheless it is food for thought!

Fasting and dieting is good for us and this is not only because it gives us a chance to practise discipline and gain self-respect; it also gives us a chance to learn that with a correct diet we will feel better and more healthy. We can see the other side of the coin when, for example, we consider the effects of salt in the diet. Salt has become a very agreeable additive for many, but observe what it does to a person with high blood pressure. He or she becomes irritated and quarrelsome, and probably rather unpleasant.

Outwardly, we can see what is happening internally. Look at the many rheumatic and arthritic people who continue to eat pork and pork-derived foods. Maybe they also smoke and drink. The signs are visible for all to see. Of course alcohol damages the liver, but it will also accelerate the breakdown of brain cells. Physically, we can see what happens to alcoholics, but unfortunately the emotional body is even more affected. You are what you eat and you are what you drink.

When I see what happens to a highly stressed person who is prepared to accept my advice, and follow a low-stress diet, I marvel at the change this brings about, which can be quite remarkable. Similar improvements are achieved when a hypertensive patient changes to follow a rice diet. So often in counselling work with cancer patients we are left in no doubt that diet plays a significant role in this illness. A cancer cell is like a brain cell. If a cancer patient decides to take positive action against the enemy, the mind will often prove stronger than the body, and some patients then experience a welcome remission. Specific dietary advice for cancer patients can be found in my book *Cancer and Leukaemia*, and it should never be forgotten that positive action will have positive results.

Mental discipline will help us to follow some general rules that apply to everyone: leave the table before being completely satisfied and make sure that the biggest part of your diet is raw food — vegetables, grains, nuts and seeds. It is important to take time to enjoy your food. Always chew well and pay attention to the quality of food. If at all possible eat organically grown or unprocessed foods. Drink carrot juice and beetroot juice, herbal teas and bottled or mineral water. Restrict the intake of salt, sugar, saturated fats, fried foods and stimulants. Try to avoid using aluminium pots and pans, because there is a growing belief that this may be a contributory factor in the occurrence of Alzheimer's disease. Be wary of microwave cooking, because this cooking method can change the L-form of the amino acids, and, finally, be very careful with all forms of additives, preservatives and colourings.

Good rest, good food and good relaxation is the rule for life. Never mix vegetables and fruits in one meal. Eat them at separate meals or else leave a minimum of twenty minutes between eating them. The correct combination of foods is very important. Although there is a wide choice of food available, variety does not automatically lead to good nutrition, because an unbalanced diet can easily cause health problems. Until the twentieth century most people in the world spent their days engaged in physical labour, therefore they expended more energy on an average day than we are likely to nowadays. The authorities cannot agree on the optimum daily calorific intake today, although most agree that it should be somewhere in the region of 2,000–4,000 calories, depending on the kind of work we do. Nowadays we are more likely to be burdened with mental worries and our brain, in order to function well, needs food that will provide the correct brain enzymes. High-protein products will not help us to cope effectively with stress, and animal protein will actually make it worse. Vegetable protein is much more appropriate in today's environment.

In answer to the question of why allergies occur, I must answer that it is because strain and stress have diminished the effectiveness of the immune system. An allergy will alter the reaction of the body tissues to a specific condition – generally dietary or environmental – which in non-sensitive people would produce no reaction at all. Biochemically, it is individually determined that one man's meat is another's poison. It is impossible to say that there are allergy-free foods and combinations. The emphasis should therefore be placed upon whole, natural, unrefined, unpolluted foods, plus healthy digestion and assimilation. If possible, an 80 per cent raw food diet would be ideal. Detoxification of the small intestine should also be investigated. This advice applies as far as food is concerned, because allergies can also be related to many other substances, which can include synthetic materials, odours, gases and pollens.

Toxicity is an ever-growing problem and throughout the world this is mainly caused by environmental contamination, for example, by agricultural sprays, air-borne toxins, petrochemical refineries, water pollution caused by industrial discharge, synthetic materials and numerous other substances that may invade the bloodstream, lymph and tissues, including those of the brain.

It is impossible to quantify the number of allergies that exist because new influences and factors are constantly coming to light that cause incomplete breakdown of foods, resulting in impaired digestion and elimination. Allergic problems may be triggered by lack of exercise, failure to eliminate through perspiration, incorrect breathing, synthetic fibres, preservatives, artificial sweeteners, synthetic flavours, chemicals, tap water, hair dyes, under-arm deodorants – the list goes on and on. Complete escape is impossible. Compensating for what cannot be avoided is a common and sensible tactic. First look at improving the diet. Next take care of the digestion. If in doubt consider taking a vitamin supplement. Here the most obvious supplement would be vitamins C and E, because both are great detoxifiers and will also encourage cell renewal.

Life is a constant renewal of cell tissue. The nervous system, which takes the brunt of all our stresses and strains, depends on good nutrition. The life force within us is controlled and dominated by the body's ability in relation to energy exchange: positive to negative. The life force is like electricity, in that it provides us with the power to run appliances and provide light and heating for our homes. To illustrate this, the human immune system – which stands guard day and night to protect our survival on a cellular level – is chemically powered by a combination of minerals, trace elements and enzymes, each of which is predominantly positively or negatively charged. Where sodium is positive, potassium is negative, and these are electrically charged energies which attract and provide transport for the fluids outside the cell, to exchange with fluids inside the cell. When in balance and not overpowered by toxins, inter-cellular fluids will be mostly potassium dominated, as opposed to the positively charged sodium molecules and extra-cellular fluids. The external cell membranes are programmed by nature to be receptive to incoming chemicals, while the internal cell membranes are programmed oppositely. When there is insufficient inter-cellular potassium or an overabundance of extra-cellular sodium, the cells become waterlogged, with insufficient exchange and low energy potential. Life is movement and death is stasis. It is the living nervous system upon which movement depends. It is the biochemical balance within body fluids and tissues, which supply the working energy units for the body's functions and reserves, that are critical to its continual efficient operations.

I have often discussed this subject with an old friend of mine, Betty Lee Moralis, and we have exchanged material and worked on diets together, in an effort to find the positive and negative balance in the diet.

Food in general influences the brain and the emotions. Depending upon one's condition, dietary regulations can mean life and the National Association of Health Stores has published some valuable dietary advice for some of the more common allergic reactions that do indeed influence the whole body.

In the case of a milk or dairy food allergy, always read the label and note that products containing any of the following are *not* milk-free:

Curds	Lactose (milk sugar)
Lactic acid	Whey
Milk – milk solids, milk protein	Lactose – reduced cow's milk

NB Calcium or magnesium caseinate supplements (casein is the main protein present in milk) should be avoided, and it should be noted that many tablets contain lactose.

It is useful to know which non-dairy (cow's milk) replacement foods are available:

Soya milk	Non-dairy soya-based brown rice puddings
Soya ice-cream	
Frozen goat's milk	Non-dairy soya-based or carob chocolates
Spray-dried goat's milk	
UHT goat's milk	Soya yoghurt
Baking powder	Soya desserts
Sunflower margarine	Soya margarine
Soya cheese (without casein)	Soya cheese spreads
Tofu dressing and dip	Salad cream-style dressing
Mayonnaise-style dressing, egg-free	Non-dairy spreads, carob

Coeliac disease develops from a sensitivity to the wheat protein gluten and similar proteins in rye, oats and barley. As a consequence of the illness, the absorptive surface of the small intestine changes to prevent the normal uptake of nutrients and a number of nutrient deficiency disorders may develop. Exclusion, usually for life, of wheat, oats, rye and barley permits the small intestine to function satisfactorily. Wheat can carry a high percentage of contaminants. Non-organic wheat can contain artificial fertilisers, herbicides, pesticides and fungicides, although organic wheat should not be affected.

When food shopping, remember to take nothing for granted: always ask first. A coeliac patient must be absolutely sure. Reading the label is sometimes no guarantee, for example in products containing spices as wheat flour is sometimes used as a base for mixing spices more evenly. Truly gluten-free products are clearly marked as such, in order to prevent mistakes.

Dietary fibre is a necessary part of a healthy diet. It has long been recognised that the benefits of food comprise more than just its nutrients. Dietary fibre is difficult to describe as it is really a mixture of material derived from plants that is not digestable by the enzymes in the human digestive tract, but is broken down in the bowel through the action of microbes which still cause it to ferment. While dietary fibre is thought to contain no nutrients for humans, it still has an essential task to perform.

There are two types of fibre: insoluble and soluble. Insoluble dietary fibre, found in wholegrain cereals and pulses (peas, beans and lentils), absorbs water in the large intestine to produce softer, bulkier stools. Insoluble fibre increases the time foods spend in the stomach, thereby permitting digestion to occur at a slightly more leisurely pace and slowing the rise in blood sugar. Transit time, the period between eating and excretion, is reduced by insoluble dietary fibre. Soluble fibre (found in oats, fruits and vegetables) may act to lower the cholesterol level.

A diet high in insoluble dietary fibre prevents constipation by promoting the formation of soft, bulky stools which may be passed without straining. It is thought that diverticular disease, where small pockets balloon out from the walls of the bowels, may be a consequence of years of straining to pass small, hard stools. Dietary fibre prevents this, and may also be a major factor in the prevention of piles (haemorrhoids) and certain life-threatening intestinal conditions.

Gall bladder disease most frequently occurs in overweight women. It may be characterised by localised inflammation or gallstones that require treatment. Weight loss is generally beneficial, as is the avoidance of irregular, large, high-fat meals. Eating little and often and ensuring meals are high in dietary fibre and low in fat can be helpful. Knowledge of the dangers, and what the alternatives are, is important.

Non-fibre foods	Fibre-rich foods
Butter	Brown rice
Cheese	Crispbread
Coffee	Fresh fruit
Eggs	Grains, e.g. millet, barley, wheat
Fish	Porridge oats
Fruit juice	Muesli
Herbal teas	Nuts
Margarine	Pulses
Meat	Seeds
Milk	Soya flour

Oils, e.g. sunflower, olive
Rye flour
Sago
Soya milk
Tapioca
Tofu
Water
Wine
Yoghurt

Wild rice
Wholemeal bread
Wholemeal flour
Vegetables

Always include as many vegetables and fresh fruit in the diet as possible. If you feel hungry between meals reach for a piece of fruit. Reduce your intake of food that is highly processed, high in sugar and made of non-wholemeal flour.

The other day I again looked into an old book entitled *Old Age Deferred*, which was written in 1910 by the Austrian physician, Dr Anhalt Lorant. Early this century he was already advocating certain dietary restrictions, and he especially mentioned sugar and meat. It was illuminating to read this account of how the nervous system is influenced by the eating of meat. Dr Lorant wrote that he had noticed that nervous disorders were more frequent after eating meat, and that more cases of neurasthenia and hysteria were diagnosed among meat eaters than among vegetarians. Meat can produce a high level of toxins and exert a strain on the vital organs, such as the thyroid gland, the liver, the kidneys and the pancreas. He maintained that meat can cause gout and arteriosclerosis and can also cause cancer. Meat can adversely influence a diabetic, and the viscosity of blood is increased and the circulation reduced. Toxins from constipated bowels inflict further strain on the kidneys where there is a high meat intake. Poultry causes these problems to a lesser degree, while fish, as a protein-deliverer, is by far the best option.

More education is necessary on this very important subject. Alexis Carrel, a one-time Nobel prize winner, is known to have said: 'Unless the doctors of today become the dieticians of tomorrow, the dieticians of today will become the doctors of tomorrow.'

24

A Healthy Metabolism

There are many forms of metabolic imbalance, as for example there are many kinds of diabetes. Any kind of metabolic imbalance should be looked at from all aspects: mental, physical and emotional. In the preceding chapter on food I concentrated on the dangers of specific foods, while in this chapter I want to point out the dangers of over-eating in general, which is bound to result in a metabolic imbalance.

Every day I see patients with metabolic problems, and many have brought these upon themselves with the wrong kind of food, and find themselves in a situation they would dearly like to escape from. I don't think that anyone can give a realistic estimate of the millions of pounds that are spent annually on slimming clinics, diets and exercises. Yet in most cases all that is needed is will power. Every ounce of food or drink we eat must be digested, absorbed and then eliminated. Much of the food we eat nowadays contains little goodness and thus its only function is to ensure a fat future. Many people with an imbalance in the three bodies have suffered from over-eating. In my book *Realistic Weight Control* I have outlined a number of many different approaches to overcoming excess weight in a healthy way. Those people who have taken the trouble are generally those who are successful. One must always believe that it can be done. There is, however, a simple definition of weight control, summed up in two small sentences: 'I think . . .' and 'I feel . . .'.

If we think about it we probably will admit that we know we should not eat so much, yet if we follow our feelings, we will probably have that other chocolate and worry about it later. Metabolic imbalances and weight problems account for a great deal of frustration, and so very quickly we reach the conclusion that we can no longer be bothered and just eat. We have to adapt the control system and see the mind as a computer: for the desired output the machine should be correctly programmed. Discipline and self-respect are essential. Keep the goal in mind and realise how much better we will feel and look. It is tremendously helpful to visualise this in the mind.

I grew up during the Second World War and in those days I never saw anyone who was overweight. It is will power that controls our house of health, because it is built on the foundation of healthy nourishment and not on obesity. Too many people have health problems which are caused by eating disorders. If we take a positive interest and discipline ourselves, we can make sure that we will reach that goal.

This is the reason why we have a slimming clinic on our premises, where people are not only helped with dietary advice, but where we also use acupressure treatment to help our patients by speeding up the metabolism, so that food is more quickly digested and eliminated. Some time ago I came across the following definition of weight problems, which certainly identifies and confirms the presence of the three bodies:

Causes
Eating more food than is needed
Insufficient exercise

External factors
Appearance
Persuasion of advertising
Pace of life
Giving up something
Marriage
Confusion
Habit
Social eating

Internal factors
No will power
No self-control
No patience
Boredom
Loneliness
Negative state of mind
Fear, worry and anxiety

Emotions
Eating for comfort
Self-indulgence
Wrong mental attitude

Insecurity
After eating still not feeling satisfied
Mastered by and not master of stomach
Temptation
Compulsion

There are numerous diets to choose from, but none will be successful unless we are determined to adhere to it. We must also always bear in mind the need to follow a *healthy* diet so that we do not cause any further damage through malnutrition.

Over the years I have worked at, and perfected, the formulation of a sensible slimming diet, and I know from experience that if my patients strictly adhere to this diet they will be successful in their attempts to reduce weight. With mental determination it is not difficult to reach that goal. The diet is outlined below.

Auchenkyle Slimming Diet
NB The secret of success with this diet, as with all diets, is to carefully weigh all your food. All soups must be made using stock cubes and vegetables only. Cream soups may be made using part of the daily milk allowance.

Daily allowances
½ pint fresh or 1 pint skimmed milk or 2 cartons plain yoghurt; 3 oz wholemeal bread; 4 oz meat, or 6 oz fish, or 4 oz smoked fish, or 5 oz chicken; 3 portions of fruit.

Weekly allowances
4 oz butter or margaraine, or 8 oz 'Gold'; 8 oz cheese; up to 7 eggs.

Exchanges for 1 oz bread
3 oz potatoes; crispbread, crackers, or water biscuits, or 2 plain biscuits; 1 oz breakfast cereal of any sort, but not sugar-coated; 1 oz porridge, cooked weight; 2 dessertspoons of cooked rice.

Variety is the spice of life
Meat: 4 oz daily, cooked in any way, except fried: beef, corned beef, kidney, lamb, liver, mutton, tongue, tripe, sweetbreads, veal

Fish: 6 oz daily (4 oz smoked), cooked in any way, except fried: crab, cod, haddock, halibut, hake, herring, kippers, lobster, ling, mackerel, mussels, oysters, pilchards, prawns, salmon, sardine, shrimps, trout, tuna

Poultry/Game: 5 oz daily, cooked in any way, except fried: chicken, turkey, rabbit, grouse, pheasant, venison

Eggs: 1 medium egg daily (optional), cooked in any way, except fried

Cheese: 1oz daily of any of the following, except cottage cheese: Caerphilly, Camembert, Cheddar, Cheshire, cottage (4 oz), Danish blue, Edam, Gruyère, Leicester, Parmesan, Roquefort, Stilton, Wensleydale, smoked Austrian

Vegetables: No restrictions: artichokes, asparagus, aubergines, bean sprouts, Brussels sprouts, beetroot, broccoli, cabbage (any type), cauliflower, celery, carrots, cress, cucumber, courgettes, chicory, leeks, lettuce, marrow, mushrooms, onions, peppers, pimentoes, parsnip, pickles, parsley, French and runner beans, radish, swede, spring onions, spinach, tomatoes

In moderation: avocado, baked beans (3–5 oz), broad beans, butter beans, haricot beans, chickpeas, peas, sweetcorn

Fruit: 3 portions daily from:

apple – 1 average	peach – 1 average
apricots – 2 fresh	pear – 1 average
banana – 1 small	pineapple – 1 slice fresh
blackberries – 4 oz	plums – 2 fresh
cooking apple – 1 large	pomegranate – 1 small
cherries – 4 oz	prunes – 6 stewed
dates – 1 oz	raisins – 1 oz
damsons – 10	raspberries – 5 oz
gooseberries – 10	rhubarb – 5 oz
grapefruit – half	strawberries – 5 oz
grapes – 3 oz	sultanas – 1 oz
melon – 1 average slice	tangerines, etc. – 2
orange – 1 average	unsweetened juice – 4 fl oz

Drinks: Tea, Russian tea, herbal tea, coffee, Bovril, Oxo, Marmite, soda water, lemon juice, tomato juice, water, Energen 1 Cal, slimline soft drinks, low-calorie tonic

Seasonings: Salt, pepper, vinegar, mustard, lemon juice, herbs, spices, Worcester sauce

NB Your daily allowance must be consumed within a period of twenty-four hours.
Eat your weekly allowance within one week.
You may eat as often as you like within your allowance. However, you must *not* eat fewer than three meals a day.

If the thyroid and the ovaries are out of balance this can often express itself in a weight problem. In such cases four Kelpasan tablets should be taken first thing in the morning, or some *Ovarium*. Another herbal remedy, SLM Formula, is especially suitable for more persistent weight problems. Always bear in mind that obesity is not only an external matter, but it can cause diabetes or high blood sugar.

In Chapter 8 I recounted my own experience of diabetes, and explained about some of the remedies that can help counter this problem. Dia-Kamp has also been of great use in some of the more severe cases of diabetes I have been asked to treat. Please note that I do not recommend refusing the doctors' prescription for tablets or insulin, but when introducing this programme, most doctors or specialists who supervise the treatment of a diabetic patient will be only too happy to reduce the medication that needs to be taken daily. It is important to study carefully the entire diabetic spectrum to discover why diabetes is so much on the increase. Perhaps it is because of increased sugar intake, combined with stress, that diabetes figures are growing, all over the world. I have seen it clearly in the years I worked in my clinic in Northern Ireland. During the twenty-five-year reign of conflict in that country, the incidence of diabetes, cancer and other serious degenerative diseases, has greatly increased. Stress-related circumstances have to be watched carefully, and support is necessary.

The condition hypoglycaemia, with its insulin excess, and the hormonal disturbances that cause the condition, is the opposite of diabetes. This can be controlled with a healthy diet, by monitoring the carbohydrate intake. The usual advice, especially for pre-menstrual and menopausal women, is to eat regular small meals every three hours, and take the excellent remedy Normoglycaemia. This unique formula also supplies Glucose Tolerance Factor (GTF) with other nutrients involved in the maintenance of normal blood sugar levels. The Women's Nutritional Advisory service has found that women may have an extra 'sweet tooth' before their periods and they recommend that the nutrients in Normoglycaemia may help maintain normal blood sugar levels and thereby help them to keep their sweet tooth in check. If there is adrenal dysfunction the stress response is often astonishing, and various exercises may have to be introduced to help overcome this condition.

Metabolic bone diseases, such as osteoporosis and osteomalacia, can be averted or better managed with some wonderful remedies such as GS-Komplex and Osteo-Prime. Imbalances are gaining the upper hand, for example in metabolic liver diseases and in excessive cholesterol production. Essential fatty acids and free radicals play a significant role in metabolic imbalances affecting cholesterol problems, diabetes mellitus, and diabetes nephropathy.

It is important that we realise what is bound to happen if we do not pay attention to our weight. An American scientist, Beall, calculated that every pound of fat requires five to six miles of blood vessels to supply it, and that a man who is 30 lb overweight is carrying twenty-five miles of excessive blood vesssels with a resulting strain upon his circulation. As we lengthen our waist line, we shorten our life line. This is not just a scare story, but these are the facts of which we should be aware, as being overweight can cause serious medical problems.

It always saddens me to see patients with anorexia or bulimia. Anorexia nervosa is a weight condition where all three bodies of man are very much involved. When one is underweight excessive destruction of body tissue takes place. Like anorexics, I do not like obesity, but tissue damage caused by under-nourishment is equally dangerous. With most anorexic patients I have treated, it has taken a long time for them to understand this, and to save them from gradual, but certain degeneration. There are some excellent remedies to maintain the balance of the metabolic system: the remedy *Centaurium* has proved successful in many cases. Supplementary vitamins, minerals and trace elements will certainly not make the anorexic patient overweight. Such supplements will help to control the body weight, but also to restore balance to the mental, physical and emotional bodies.

The mineral zinc is very important in the treatment of anorexia and bulimia, and I often prescribe a zinc supplement. This mineral assists in the release of carbon-dioxide into the blood, and together with mangenese, zinc helps bone formation and strength. It balances cholesterol deposits, prevents white spots on the nails, regulates menstruation, encourages eye muscle contractibility, activates enzymes, helps to form insulin, aids wound healing, and can restore the senses of taste and smell. Zinc and chromium are great partners if they are used together in the treatment of some of these very difficult problems.

Alkaline/acid metabolic disturbances are more common today, and this can be seen in the ever-increasing incidence of rheumatism and arthritis, as it is thought that these conditions are partially caused by an acid-alkaline imbalanced diet. From urine samples of patients with arthritis, rheumatism, psoriasis, eczema and duodenal or peptic ulcers, we see that there is always an over-acidity in the system, and a balanced diet is important for treating most metabolic general conditions. Diets should be considered on an individual basis, but often by cutting out the acid-forming products, such as anything from the pig, citrus fruits, coffee, tea and chocolate, nicotine and alcohol, the goal moves within our reach. Mentally this needs adjustment, as much as, if not more so, than physically.

The other day I was called across the street by an acquaintance who asked me to come and say hello to his wife. This relatively young woman was in a wheelchair, crippled with arthritis. With tears in her eyes, she said that she regretted that she had not listened to me, but she had been unable to give up the foods she enjoyed and yet it was the food that had been her destruction. Is it worth while continuing to indulge in the foods we love so much, without thinking about their effects on our body and our health? I told her that it was never too late to adjust the diet and to introduce the nutrients and foods that will assist in a better acid/alkaline balance.

It is interesting to read about the new development and research that is done with amino acid sugars, even where the collagen under the skin is seriously damaged. With remedies such as Armax and GS-Komplex damage can often be repaired. Female patients, because of a pre-menopausal condition, may become arthritic, caused by imbalances in the hormonal system. With dietary control and natural remedies much can be achieved to control or rectify these conditions.

There has been a lot of publicity regarding the treatment of osteoarthritis using different forms of cartilage products, but none has received such outstanding and reproducible results in clinical studies as glucosamine sulphate (GS). This is a naturally occurring aminomonosaccharide found in joint cartilage, consisting of glucose and sulphur. In an update on a research project into the usefulness of GS it was stated that osteoarthrosis is a classic example where current medical treatment suppresses symptoms. Since conventional treatment does not address the underlying cause it actually promotes the disease process. The use of GS is an example of how a natural substance improves a condition by addressing the underlying cause and supports the body's ability to heal itself.

On the subject of metabolic imbalance I must again stress the point mentioned in the context of the building of our house of health. The main materials used for building the house are essential fatty acids, hence the reason I have frequently mentioned Evening Primrose Oil. Glucose and other essential fatty acids are also requirements, as are vitamins, minerals and trace elements, amino acids, enzymes and oxygen. All these nutrients relate to the five important pillars of the house of health: nutrition, digestion, elimination, circulation and relaxation. A chemical balance will be found if these five pillars rest upon a sound foundation. These nutrients will help the house to withstand internal and external attacks.

25

That's Health

As I write this last chapter, I am sitting about 500 yards away from a house I last visited on 16 August 1960. Every time I pass that house I think of the determination I felt when I closed the door there at noon on that day. I was called to that house by the provincial Inspector of Health. Two other doctors were summoned along with me, and all three of us were instructed to immediately cease work at the very first clinic in the Netherlands established to practice naturopathic medicine, according to the principles of Dr Alfred Vogel. One of the doctors withdrew, while the other and I left with more determination than ever because we knew how many hospital beds were occupied unnecessarily, how many doctors had their injections prepared before even having seen the patient, and were well aware of the tremendous turmoil that reigned in the world of medicine. Nevertheless, the Inspector of Health was required to follow the guidelines as laid down by the Ministry of Health, excluding any practice of alternative medicine. I could see that the health of the population was deteriorating and, although young and inexperienced, I knew that there was more that we could do to help people. This happened when I was the first managing director of Biohorma, which is now a thriving business in the Netherlands, with a workforce of some three hundred people, helping so many who previously had been solely dependent on drugs. I was determined not to give up, but to keep fighting, even although I was threatened that my certificates would be confiscated, and it was possible I could be arrested.

How that picture has changed today. I have seen the tremendous growth in the numbers of doctors who, alongside conventional medicine, also practise some form of complementary medicine, which is now permitted by a much more flexible system.

I often think of the time I visited a colleague of mine in prison, and we talked about Copernicus, who shattered all the beliefs of the scientific establishment in the sixteenth and seventeenth centuries, with his views on the solar system. At that time he was considered to be insane, but now we know that he was an enlightened visionary, whose principles have since been proved to be correct. I am quite sure of our Creator's intentions when he promised that man would be given herbs for healing and food to exist. Nature provides everything for our needs and the more natural we can keep nature's gifts the better.

The first chapter of this book I entitled 'What is Health?', in contrast to the title of the present chapter 'That's Health'. Since 1960 I have never ceased in my efforts to spread the message of how natural medicine can be used to ease human suffering, and thankfully I have been joined in this effort by many others. This movement has gained in strength all over the world, finding the ear of hundreds of thousands of people, and also with much help from people in the established medical world. The World Health Organisation (WHO) has the laudable aim 'Health for All by the year 2000'. Will it ever happen? In their definition the WHO states that health is a state of physical, mental and social well-being, and not merely the absence of disease or debility. Do we really believe that health lies within our reach if we continue to poison the world by spraying chemical compounds onto the soil, and lacing our food with chemical preservatives and artificial colourings? A few years ago I had the honour of being invited by the WHO to open a major health conference, which that year was held in a developing country where the staple diet was rice. On that visit I realised that some of our Western habits were making rapid inroads there, because I could not fail to notice that the youngsters were walking about with cans of fizzy drinks, eating chocolate bars and crisps. I then began to doubt whether health for all by the end of the twentieth century was indeed within our reach. Rice, which is the staple food of that country, was rotting in their stores. Didn't they realise that rice has all the qualities required to balance one's health? We must stop and think about what we are doing.

Life is a constant renewal of cells, and in trying to understand the meaning of health, if we fail to consider the life processes which maintain the living organisms, we do not gain anything. We need to have some knowledge of scientific principles to understand these, but nature is simple and nature will tell us by intuition what must be done. The scientific concept of health is that of a living organism, continually in balance. Health is not a stable condition like a solid superstructure on a concrete foundation, but rather a process in unceasing motion wherein the organism successfully adapts and compensates in order to survive. I like the expression of my great friend Dr Allan, who said that the whole process is dynamic equilibrium. The whole world today is living continuously below the level of our powers of observation, within the billions of cells which form the smallest unit of structure in our bodies. Sudden upsets of that equilibrium of the chemistry of cells through the ingestion of toxic substances can suddenly change the condition of the body from health to illness.

As living organisms, we move continuously and irreversibly through moments, hours, days, months and years, but never more than a moment at a time, responding and reacting to external and internal stimuli, reflecting our own individual habit patterns. The health of every individual from a physical standpoint depends upon how well the body adapts itself to internal and external environmental changes, to injuries, to stress and strain, and to the exposure to toxic and disease producing agents. If we look at health for the future, it is a matter of positive action. In regretting the past we forfeit the future. In this modern age of nuclear energy and other innovations, we must correspond to the scientific facts and learn to correctly interpret the word science. In the dictionary I read the definition of the word 'science' is to discover the secrets of nature and make these available to man. The term health is better understood within the concept of dynamic equilibrium.

This morning I received a letter written by a young man who expressed his sadness about earthly pollution, dreaming of one day living in a world free of pollution, and no longer having to witness the destruction of the world as we know it. He writes that mankind has destroyed its own health and questions what has happened to the basic laws of nature. He idealistically imagines living in a world where love reigns and everything is in harmony. He also writes that his objective mind, his subjective mind and his subconscious mind are often influenced by thoughts that are taking the discussion away from a universal mind. I had great sympathy with the writer of this letter and in my answer I advised him to use visualisation techniques to influence the conscious mind with pictures of what can be, looking at the better things in life and ways to improve one's own life, in order to try and improve our existence in the world. I also mentioned in my letter that it was my firm belief that God never intended us to be sick or to feel only half alive.

In the United States I have heard it said that one-third of the American people are physically, mentally or emotionally impaired. These figures were released by the Health Education Committee. The other day *The Observer* featured an article where it claimed that British industry loses an estimated eighteen million man hours every year due to psychiatric illness, compared to four million caused by strike action. We certainly cannot afford to be sick, and we should be getting on with life, enjoying it to the full, as there is so much to do. There are no excuses for feeling only half alive. We need to learn how to really live and discover a positive mental attitude that spells HEALTH. Fresh air and physical exercise will help to recharge the body aided by breathing exercises. Plenty of rest and sleep is necessary when life is lived at today's hectic pace.

After a recent public lecture I was handed a sheet of paper with the seven basic rules of radiant health and when I was preparing this chapter I realised that these were most appropriate.

1. Quit worrying, arguing, bickering. Maintain a tranquil mind and a positive attitude.
2. Be sure you have a balanced diet of natural foods. Learn the value of drinking plenty of water and fasting, and of avoiding constipation.
3. Remember that cleanliness is vital to good health and that suitable clothing is necessary.
4. Derive the maximum benefit from sunshine and fresh air.
5. Plan a programme of regular sufficient exercise.
6. Let your body recuperate from work and play by proper sleep and rest as God intended.
7. Take care of the healthy body you are building. Avoid bodily injury.

Sometimes we forget what health is all about. We forget that if we live in tune with nature it will always be our best friend. The other day I met a young man, who was very capable and with an excellent brain, but somehow he had lost his zest for life. He came to see me while his mind was very disturbed and he was most unhappy about events that had happened recently. He was in such a depressed and desperate state that I had to give him some Emergency Essence, a combination remedy of several herbs with typical characteristics to deal with trauma. Emotional trauma had triggered physical trauma, where with an accumulation of many factors, he had to discover the original cause. I showed him a card on which I had listed a number of diseases I had studied. When I mentioned the term 'Functional auto-suggestions', he looked up and I showed him that this was known in medicine as accounting for 80 per cent of all disease. He admitted that all causes of disease, as mentioned in the table on page 230, applied to him:

Organic poisons (15%)	Structural trauma (5%)	Functional auto-suggestion (80%)
Germs, filth, etc.	Shock	Genetic tendencies
Excess food	Falls	Intense talk
Excess drink	Accidents	Vibration of disease
Burns	Sprains	Emotional stress
Pollen		

Once he started to talk he began to understand some of his problems without any prompting from me. He said that he had to learn to think more positively, and also that he had to think and act as a man. Possibly because he had lived through such a traumatic period, he asked me a strange question: 'Do you really think that God still loves me?' I replied that there was an enormous difference between divine and human love. The latter means that people love, not because of what they are, but because of the recipient. However, God loves not because of what we are, but because of what He is. With His great wisdom and love God will restore our health – mentally, physically and emotionally. Our Creator did more than create heaven and earth; He wants to personally guide and sustain us whilst we are on this planet, where we are just a minute part of that great miracle. With the power of that knowledge we can overcome many things by using this divine force to restore the life force within us. If we think of that great wonder that is Life, and understand that true sense of creation, we will then motivate ourselves to appreciate this power, recognising that we play a small role in that great universe.

I am writing this chapter in the Netherlands, while several million people are being evacuated because of the very serious danger of flooding. Because of exceptional rainfall and floods in Germany and Belgium, the dikes of the main rivers in the Netherlands are in danger of bursting, the more so because most of the country lies below sea level. In 1953 there were major floods, when a large part in the west of the Netherlands was flooded, costing the lives of some two thousand people, and many more heads of livestock. I have spoken to many people who lost everything they had in those floods, not only material possessions, but also friends and relatives. Each of them, at some time, has admitted that the great lesson they learned was the value of life, and that, temporarily, the true value of their worldly possessions definitely came second when their lives, and the lives of their families, were in danger.

I will never forget the story I was told by an elderly miner in Scotland. This man told me that once he was trapped underground with twelve of his colleagues. Without light or food, they were completely isolated for days. They tried to comfort each other, each recognising that the chance of survival was becoming less by the minute. He told me that he remembered a prayer from school, which he repeated over and over again:

Out of the depths I cry to Thee, oh Lord.
Lord, hear my voice.
Let Thy ears be attentive to the voice of my supplications.

He admitted that he repeated this text, in the darkness, every time he was unable to put aside the realisation of how precarious their situation was. He said that no matter how long he lived, he would never forget when they saw the first ray of light. Love had grown between him and his colleagues, and that love would last forever. Love is still one of the best remedies for health. Universal love is the only commandment in the New Testament, yet is sorely lacking in today's society. Often the lack of this love is the cause of disturbance in the three bodies of man. Disturbance is disharmony. Harmony of these three bodies is essential and a positive outlook: *That's Health.*

In this book I would like to say goodbye to all my readers with some daily exercises I try to practise as often as I can:

1. Relax: I have cast my burden.
2. Stretch: My arms to catch the bounty that is mine.
3. Inhale: The one perfect life, breathe in beauty.
4. Exhale: Critical and negative thoughts.
5. Brain exercise: Think only constructive thoughts.
6. Eye exercise: See only perfection in others.
7. Ear exercise: Listen for the voice of the Innate.
8. Facial exercise: Smile – smile – smile.
9. Tongue exercise: Speak kindness.
10. Head exercise: Broadcast thoughts of love.
11. Leg exercise: Walk fearlessly in the path God directs.
12. Soul exercise: Commune with the Innate within.

These exercises will give you all you require: *HEALTH – WEALTH – HAPPINESS.*

Glossary of Remedies and Suppliers

Acidophilus Extra	Nature's Best
Acne-Zyme	Enzymatic Therapy
Aesculaforce	Bioforce
Alchemilla Complex	Bioforce
Alfalfa	Nature's Best
Aquaflow	Enzymatic Therapy
Araniforce	Auchenkyle
Argentum nit	Homoeopathic remedy
Armax	Enzymatic Therapy
Arnica	Bioforce
Arterioforce	Bioforce
Asthma drops	Bioforce
Atropa	Homoeopathic remedy
Aurum	Homoeopathic remedy
Avena sativa	Bioforce
Belladonna D4	Homoeopathic remedy
Boldocynara	Bioforce
Bronchosan	Bioforce
CPS	Enzymatic Therapy
Cardiaforce	Bioforce
Centaurium	Bioforce
Cerebrum	Auchenkyle
Chelate Formula	Nature's Best
Chem-Ex	Enzymatic Therapy
Chromium	Nature's Best
Co-Enzyme Q10	Nature's Best
Cocculus	Bioforce
Crataegisan	Bioforce
Cystoforce	Bioforce
DGL	Enzymatic Therapy
Devil's Claw	Bioforce

Dia-Comp	Enzymatic Therapy
Diabetes Komplex	Bioforce
Diabetisan	Bioforce
DLPA Complex	Nature's Best
Dormeasan	Bioforce
Echinaforce	Bioforce
Euphrasiasan	Bioforce
Evening Primrose	Nature's Best
Galeopsis	Bioforce
Garlic capsules	Nature's Best
Ginkgo biloba	Bioforce
Ginsavita	Bioforce
Golden Grass Tea	Bioforce
GS1000	Enzymatic Therapy
GTF Chromium	Nature's Best
Hair and Skin Capsules	Enzymatic Therapy
Hamamelis	Bioforce
Harpagophytum	Bioforce
Health Insurance Plus	Nature's Best
Hepar sulph.	Homoeopathic remedy
Herbal Health Complex	Enzymatic Therapy
Herbamare	Bioforce
Herpilyn	Hadley Wood Healthcare
Hyperisan	Bioforce
Ignatia	Homoeopathic remedy
Imperarthritica	Bioforce
Imuno-Strength	Nature's Best
Jayvee tablets	Nature's Best
Kelpasan	Bioforce
Lachesis	Bioforce
Linoforce	Bioforce
Lycopus eur.	Homoeopathic remedy
Lympho-Clear	Enzymatic Therapy
Magnesium phos.	Homoeopathic remedy
Marum verum	Bioforce
Maxi-Hair	Nature's Best
Milk Thistle Extract	Enzymatic Therapy
Molkosan	Bioforce
Nat mur.	Homoeopathic remedy
Natrium sulph.	Homoeopathic remedy

Nephrosolid	Bioforce
Nettle Lotion	Bioforce
Neuroforce	Bioforce
Normoglycaemia	Nature's Best
Nux vomica	Homoeopathic remedy
Occulosan	Auchenkyle
Onion Hair Lotion	Bioforce
Oral Nutrient Chelate	Enzymatic Therapy
Osteo-Care	Vitabiotics
Osteo-Prime	Enzymatic Therapy
Ovarium 3	Homoeopathic remedy
Papayaforce	Bioforce
Petasan	Bioforce
Phosphorus D6	Homoeopathic remedy
Phyto-Biotic	Enzymatic Therapy
Plantago	Bioforce
Playfair	Nature's Best
Podophyllum pelt.	Homoeopathic remedy
Pollinosan	Bioforce
Poho oil	Bioforce
Priorin	Auchenkyle
Propolis Wart Tincture	Hadley Wood Healthcare
Prostabrit	Britannia Health Products
Prostasan	Bioforce
Protein Deficiency Formula	Nature's Best
Rasayana Course	Bioforce
Rhus tox.	Homoeopathic remedy
Rubiaforce	Bioforce
Santasapina	Bioforce
Selenium	Nature's Best
Seven Herb Cream	Bioforce
Sina D4	Homoeopathic remedy
Sinu-Check	Enzymatic Therapy
Sinus Formula	Bioforce
SLM Formula	Bioforce
SNS Formula	Bioforce
Solidago	Bioforce
Spigaelia	Homoepathic remedy
Spilanthes	Bioforce
Spring Cleansing Course	Bioforce

St. John's wort	Bioforce
Stay Calm	Montana
Temoe Lawak	Auchenkyle
Thuja	Homoeopathic remedy
Tormentavena	Bioforce
Trocamare	Bioforce
Urticalcin	Bioforce
Usneasan	Bioforce
Viola tricolor	Bioforce
Viral-Plex	Enzymatic Therapy
Viscum album	Bioforce
Vision Essentials	Enzymatic Therapy
Vitaforce	Bioforce
Vyr-Brit	Britannia Health
Zincum valerianum	Auchenkyle

Useful Addresses

Auchenkyle, Southwoods Road, Troon, Ayrshire KA10 7EL

Bach Flower Remedies, Unit 6, Suffolk Way, Abingdon, Oxon OX14 5JX

Bioforce UK Ltd, Olympic Business Park, Dundonald, Ayrshire KA2 9BE

Bioforce Canada Ltd, 11 German Street, Newmarket, Ontario L3Y 7V1

Bioforce USA Ltd, Kinderhook, New York, NY, USA

Britannia Health Products Ltd, Forum House, Brighton Road, Redhill, Surrey RH1 6YS

British Acupuncture Association, 34 Alderney Street, London SW1V 4EU

Enzymatic Therapy, Hadley Wood Healthcare, 67a Beech Hill, Hadley Wood, Barnet, Herts EN4 0JW

Enzymatic Therapy, PO Box 22310, Green Bay W1 54305, USA

General Council and Register of Naturopaths, Frazer House, 6 Netherhall Gardens, London NW3 5RR

General Council and Register of Osteopaths, 56 London Street, Reading, Berks RG1 4SQ

Hadley Wood Healthcare, 67a Beech Hill, Hadley Wood, Barnet,

Herts EN4 0JW

Montana, Hadleigh Wood Healthcare, 67a Beech Hill, Hadley Wood, Barnet, Herts

Nature's Best, Dept. HT01, 1 Lamberts Road, Tunbridge Wells, Kent TH2 3EQ

A. Nelson & Co. Ltd, 5 Endeavour Way, Wimbledon, London SW19 9UH

Obbekjaers, 209 Blackburn Road, Wheelton, Chorley, Lancs

Sans Soucis, Hadley Wood Healthcare, 67a Beech Hill, Hadley Wood, Barnet, Herts EN4 0JW